Aromatherapy Pocketbook

The *Aromatherapy Pocketbook* overflows with facts, tips, and recipes, including:

- Answers to the most-asked questions about aromatherapy.

- A-Z list of the basic oils, including botanical family, principle components, climate of origin, oil extraction, blending class, history and lore, therapeutic properties, planet, and elemental correspondences.

- Instructions for blending essential oils, making botanical perfumes, and creating personal fragrances.

- The essentials of natural skin care to clean, nourish, moisturize, stimulate, and heal the complexion.

- Instructions for creating a medical travel/first aid kit, as well as a list of common ailments and how to treat them.

- Fascinating case histories of healing.

- How to combine the vibrational energies of natural stones with scents.

About the Author

Kendra Grace was born in Bahia, Brazil, and came to the United States as an exchange student twenty-five years ago. She lives in Northern California with her husband and their three daughters. Kendra recently completed a trip around the world producing a documentary film called *Aromatherapy Journeys,* about the production of the essential oils from flowers.

Kendra was introduced to aromatherapy fifteen years ago by Dr. Kurt Schnaubelt of the Pacific Institute of Aromatherapy in San Rafael, California. Ever since then she has been devoted to the study and practice of this exciting new science.

Using her multifaceted background developed from her extensive research in both aromatic plants, natural stones, and the healing arts, Kendra developed a synergy concept, realized in a line of subtle aromatherapy jewelry known worldwide as Aromajewels, combining the power of essential oils with the energetic influence of crystals and gems. These jewels are utilized in vibrational medicine.

Aromatherapy Pocketbook

Kendra Grace

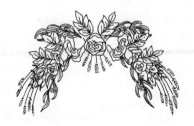

1999
Llewellyn Publications
St. Paul, Minnesota   55164-0383, U.S.A.

SECOND EDITION
First printing, 1999
First edition, 1994

Cover design by Lisa Novak
Cover photo by Mike Chase
Botanical illustrations by Carrie Westfall
Facial illustrations by Kendra Grace
Editing and interior design by Astrid Sandell

Library of Congress Cataloging-in-Publications Data
Grace, Kendra
    [Aromatherapy pocket book]
    Aromatherapy pocketbook / Kendra Grace. — 2nd ed.
        p.   cm.
    Previous ed. published as: The aromatherapy pocket book
    Includes bibliographical references.
    ISBN 1-56718-183-X (alk. paper)
    1. Aromatherapy—Handbooks, manuals, etc. I. Title.
    RM666.A68G73 1999
    615'.321—dc21   99-11966
                                                                          CIP

The written material within this book refers to historical and personal data. The author holds no claims regarding the therapeutic uses of essential oils. This book has the purpose of educating and should not be used as a substitute for traditional medical care.

Llewellyn Publications
A Division of Llewellyn Worldwide, Ltd.
P.O. Box 64383, Dept. K183-X
St. Paul, Minnesota 55164-0383

Printed in the United States of America

To Write to the Author

If you wish to contact the author or would like more information about this book, please write to the author in care of Llewellyn Worldwide, and we will forward your request. Both the author and publisher appreciate hearing from you and learning of your enjoyment of this book and how it has helped you. Llewellyn Worldwide cannot guarantee that every letter written to the author will be answered, but all will be forwarded. Please write to:

Kendra Grace
% Llewellyn Worldwide
P.O. Box 64383, Dept. K183-X
St. Paul, MN 551640-0383, U.S.A.

Please enclose a self-addressed, stamped envelope for reply, or $1.00 to cover costs. If outside U.S.A., enclose international postal reply coupon.

Dedication

This book is dedicated to the most important
women in my life:

My grandmother, Euflorsina, whose name means
of the flowers, and who was an accomplished herbalist,
by natural choice, in the remote backlands of her
farm in Bahia, Brazil.

My mother, Diva, who passed on to me my
grandmother's way, even in the midst of the
growing medical technology of the big cities.

My three daughters, Yavanna, Quendi, and
Natasha, who will undoubtedly pass on to the
future my experience of aromatherapy.

Contents

| Preface | xi |
| Acknowledgments | xiii |

1	Introduction to Aromatherapy	1
2	The Essential Oils	29
	Definitions of Therapeutic Actions	89
3	Blending Essential Oils	91
4	Cosmetic Aromatherapy	107
5	Medical Aromatherapy	143
6	Psycho-Aromatherapy	159
7	The Use of Scent in Magic	181
8	Vibrational Medicine	191

| Appendix | 229 |
| Index | 243 |

Preface

What is wonderful about aromatherapy is that you can become engaged in a relationship with the essential oils, leading to an experience that generates something unique of your self that you can share with others.

In the photograph on the cover of this book, I am holding a bouquet of roses provided by Vintage Gardens, a nursery in northern California that specializes in antique European varieties of roses. I went to them looking for a rose similar to the *Rosa damascena* of Bulgaria. What I found turned out to be quite a nice story that surprised me in a joyful way. The roses I am holding are "Autumn damask," a wonderfully fragrant variety and a cousin of the *Rosa damascena* of Bulgaria. The Autumn damask blooms in the fall, instead of the spring, as with the Bulgarian rose. The ancient Romans grew the Autumn damask for its outstanding fragrance.

Kendra Grace
Sebastopol, California

Acknowledgments

David Kent, Bette Potter for editing.

Brian Cook for information on minerals, brainstorming, and editing.

My special thanks to:

My Brazilian family, especially Ive Barbosa da Silva, my mother Diva Botelho, my father Julio Botelho, my black mama Loli, Ilma Barbosa da Silva and Emanoel da Silva, Yavanna and Quendi Cook, Mark Hill, and Katara Rae, who all played a role in helping my environment stay together while I was writing this book.

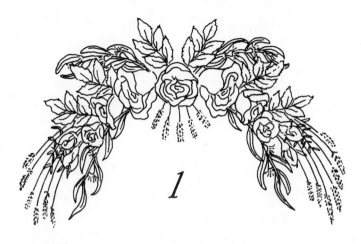

1

Introduction to Aromatherapy

The Most-Asked Questions

1. What is aromatherapy?

Aromatherapy is the art and science of using the therapeutic properties of essential oils to promote the health and well-being of the body, mind, and emotions.

2. How long has aromatherapy been used?

Aromatherapy has been used since antiquity, and records exist of its use for at least 5,000 years. In history, the Egyptians appear to be the civilization most dedicated to the art and science of aromatherapy, using incense, perfume, and cosmetics both spiritually and medicinally. We have proof of this in stone inscriptions that give us knowledge of their formulas and spiritual practices with aromatic materials. Text is also found in the vedic literature of India, dating to 4000 B.C., about the use of aromatic materials for medicine and cosmetics. This is what gave birth to a branch of the Ayurvedic System of medicine. China also has manuscripts that are as old as the vedic ones, including the Chinese medicine records of the Yellow Emperor, which describe uses for aromatic material. Mesopotamian civilizations used aromatic anointing as part of their spiritual practice. Later, Greeks and Romans, as well as the Arabian civilizations, inherited knowledge from the Egyptians and spread the use of aromatics throughout the Mediterranean region. In late A.D. 900, an Arabian doctor and philosopher named Abu Ali Ibn Sina, known in the west as "Avicenna," developed the method of distillation of essential oils as we do it today, isolating the plant's aromatic material to obtain an oil. Later, the knowledge was preserved in Europe, kept mostly by the French and used by priests, alchemists, and women and men versed in the healing arts. It is also important to remember that primitive man used fumigations—the burning of aromatic plants—which can be seen as the first use of aromatherapy.

Aromatherapy is something that has always been used, and it is very unlikely that its use will become extinct. In fact, with the refined technology we now have available, we are learning more and more about the therapeutic use of essential oils.

3. How did aromatherapy fall into obscurity after being so popular in the ancient world?

With the industrial revolution, scientific trends emerged with investigation of oils and the creation of synthetic compounds. Synthetic compounds became more prestigious, important for their "purity." It reminds me of the prestige attached to white bread during a time when the understanding of the importance of bread's fiber was lacking. Now we are examining with more care the importance of trace elements.

During the Renaissance, the use of botanical oils was still practiced by alchemists and perfumers in Europe, which went hand in hand with herbalism and medicine.

It is my belief that the development of artificial oils has produced a massive olfactory confusion, disrupting the evolution of the former knowledge, with all of its implications. During a lecture at the third annual conference of the American Aromatherapy Association, archeologist and aromatic consultant John Steele, explained from the perspective of sensorial anthropology that modern civilization is undergoing what he calls an olfactory "sensory amnesia"—which manifests as a diminished awareness of smell. I believe that synthetic molecules create a barrier in our perception of the signals we receive from nature, which we need in order to develop and realize the potential for our holistic olfactory experience.

4. *Why is aromatherapy so popular lately?*

I believe humanity is ready for gentler and more holistic ways of healing and treating the earth and the body with greater ecological awareness. People all over the world are leaning toward natural alternative forms of medicine and cosmetics.

At the turn of the millennium, modern civilization is weary and becoming increasingly mental and visual. The aromatic experience brings us down to earth and into the body, creating more balance and helping to heal stress. The pleasure that aromatherapy offers seems to be an easy route to open the mind so that significant healing can take place.

5. *What are essential oils?*

Essential oils are very volatile substances produced from botanical sources. They are the concentrates of aromatic molecules of a plant or its parts; they can be considered the hormones of the plant, as they seem to control certain functions of plant life, including the temperature and the immune system. Essential oils are also similar to a hormone in that they can stimulate or slow down biological function of cell metabolism. Many people think of essential oils as the "spirit" of the plant.

6. What does the word "botanical" mean?

Botanical is a frequently misused word that, when applied correctly, means "from plant origin." A true botanical oil has not been created by synthesis in a laboratory, but has been distilled or extracted from the plant or its parts.

7. What are essential oils made of?

Essential oils are compositions made of the basic organic elements: carbon, oxygen and hydrogen, forming alcohols, aldehydes, esters, ketones, oxides, phenols, and terpenes. An essential oil can contain between 10 and 200 components and other minor trace compounds that are very difficult to analyze. Each essential oil has a more or less complex composition. Some are very simple, as in the case of sandalwood, containing 95 percent of one compound—an alcohol called santalol—and 5 percent of combined composition.

Essential oils form very interesting and specific molecules that react against such microorganisms as bacteria and viruses. Such molecules can sometimes form a vitamin composition or a hormone-type chemical.

8. Are synthetic oils chemically the same as botanical oils?

There are chemists who like to proclaim that synthetic and botanical oils are chemically the same; however, the botanical oils have been proven by experience over thousands of years to have therapeutic or healing properties. The same cannot be said about synthetic oils. In fact, the opposite is true. (Jean Valnet, M.D., *The Practice of Aromatherapy*, p. 27.)

It is my belief that the oil from a plant that grew out of soil under sunshine and rain has an extremely different action to communicate to the human body than an oil born of laboratory synthesis. The action is unique to a botanical oil because its balance is formed out of a holistic situation.

Since our bodies are natural living organisms, it makes sense that the extract from another natural living organism would have a more harmonious and efficient interaction than it would with a synthetic compound existing under no living matrix. Can we create ocean water in the lab to be the same as the ocean?

Synthetic oils may be too "pure," too simple a composition, and not subtle enough to perform the same complex functions as botanical oils. One may say that trace elements aren't important and that they make a composition "impure"; however, it is known that if humans occupying a space shuttle mission were away from the Earth long enough, surviving solely on synthetic compounds, then trace elements would become indispensable to sustain their lives.

Why do aromatherapists speak of essential oils having life force? I think that perhaps the minute and difficult to analyze trace elements may hold that part of the composition that pertains to what we call life force. Our systems can "recognize" and respond to the living balance (the natural signals) of the botanical oils. One of the important revelations of the rediscovery of aromatherapy is the memory of essential oils as life-giving substances, which has been lost to the West since the industrial revolution.

9. Are "synthetic" and "adulterated" the same thing?

No, *synthetic* and *adulterated* are not the same thing. Some botanical oils that are available commercially—for example, eucalyptus and lavender—have been put through a number of redistillations. This process insures the so-called "purity" of the pharmaceutical and fragrance industry. For therapeutic uses, this purity actually ruins the original chemical balance of the oil, as it creates a greater percentage of its principal constituent than the original composition had. These oils are adulterated. The balance between active principal and trace elements is completely modified. Adulterated can also mean that an oil that is being sold as a pure essential oil, but has been extended with vegetable oil or diethyl phtalat. Adulteration sometimes happens even before an oil enters the commercial market; at the distillation process, other plant material can enter the distillation equipment "to fill" for a certain production that will be labeled as the principal plant being distilled.

There is also what is called "reconstruction" of oils. This occurs when some components of an essential oil are used to create a composition that imitates another oil. This is the case of a cheaper oil being used for the isolation of a component that can be used in the composition of a more expensive oil. One example of this is the component geraniol, an alcohol found both in the less expensive oil of geranium and in the expensive rose oil. Although a "reconstruction" can use components from a botanical source, the finished result is a man-made composition in imitation of an original oil.

In the case of synthetic oils, compositions can be made in the lab without using components from plant sources.

10. How can one determine if an oil has been adulterated?

To determine if an oil has been adulterated, it is first important to become familiar with essential oils from a reputable source—oils that are distributed for the aromatherapy market. (See Appendix at the end of this book.)

If you have spent a good amount of time smelling essential oils, you will soon be able to distinguish the difference between the gentle feel of essential oils, in spite of their powerful smell. Oils that are redistilled, reconstructed, or synthetic will be perceived as somewhat harsher. The more trained your nose becomes in smelling, the easier it will become to tell if the natural balance of a composition has been upset. One simple thing to remember is that essential oils do not leave an oily residue on the surface of your skin. If the oil you are testing does leave a residue, this oil has been extended with vegetable oil. Diethyl phtalat is a clear and odorless chemical commonly used to extend essential oils.

11. Are essential oils like vegetable oils?

Essential oils and vegetable oils are similar only in that they are both from plant origin. Essential oils do not consist of fatty molecules as vegetable oils do. Essential oils are aromatic and volatile, vegetable oils are not. Essential oils are volatile and evaporate rapidly, leaving no residue. Essential oils can vary in density—some have the consistency of water, others can be solid. They vary in color (clear, yellow, green, blue, orange, red, etc.) and have a powerful smell. They can be diluted in vegetable oil, alcohol, or vinegar.

12. *Can essential oils go rancid? Is there anything that can damage essential oils?*

Rancidity, which presents itself as a foul smell in vegetable oils, does not happen with essential oils. Essential oils can age as gracefully as good wines, provided that they are carefully preserved in a dark, cool place in tightly closed bottles when not in use.

Avoid exposing essential oils to direct light, heat, or contamination by another oil or substance. If these precautions have not been observed, there is the possibility that the oils can become vulnerable to change and lose their potency—their life force.

13. *How are essential oils produced?*

Steam distillation is the most common way to produce essential oils. Plant materials can be processed by hot water steam distillation in a still (an apparatus consisting of a vat, a tank for holding the plants, and another tank for producing steam from water). After essential oils are extracted from plants into the hot water, the temperature is lowered to separate the oil, which rises to the surface and is then decanted away from the water.

Cold expression can only be used in cases where the aromatic material can be easily obtained without the use of heat. All citrus oils go through this process, which extracts the oil from the rind of the fruit by mechanical pressing. In the food industry, these oils are called *essence*.

In the case of flowers so delicate that the aromatic material can be damaged by heat, the method of solvent extraction is used. Rose, orange blossom (neroli), and ylang ylang are the only flowers that can withstand the heat of steam distillation without damage, although the resulting oil's smell is not as close to the flower smell as achieved with solvent extraction.

15. Can you explain solvent extraction further?

Solvent extraction is a method that uses hydrocarbon-type solvents, products from the petro-chemical industry such as acetone, hexane, butane, and propane. It can produce a smell truer to the flowers than hot water steam distillation can. What is obtained is a creamy solid called the "concrete." This concrete contains a percentage of the flower wax that has to be further refined, and the petro-chemical solvent that has to be removed using ethanol alcohol, to produce the final substance of the process, the absolute. Absolutes can be extracted from other plant parts as well, but when it is extracted from flowers, this absolute is a precious flower oil.

16. How are concretes and absolutes used in aromatherapy?

Concretes and absolutes are produced for the fragrance industry. These oils have traces of solvent residues, which is not desirable for use in medical aromatherapy, when oils are sometimes prescribed to be taken internally.

I have used these flower oils extensively in psycho-aromatherapy, and I feel that a massage oil with a small amount of these precious flower oils does no harm. The precious flower oils have therapeutic properties as well, as the long history of their use has demonstrated.

17. How did people in the past obtain the oils from the flowers?

Oils were obtained by an old method, now abandoned, called *enfleurage*—a process using animal fat. Enfleurage consisted of placing flower petals on top of a layer of fat to saturate the fat with the aromatic material. The flowers were removed at the end of the day and a fresh layer applied, until saturation had reached desired strength. In this method, the aromatic oil would be used with the fatty base. In ancient times, aromatic oils were made by "infusion," the placement of herbs and flowers into vegetable oils. These mixtures were exposed to the sun for a period of time.

18. Is there any modern method that produces a true-to-nature smell of flowers in an oil that is also free of residue?

Extraction by liquid carbon dioxide is one modern method that produces a true smell that is also free of residue. It is performed just above room temperature. Since carbon dioxide can act as an inert gas, it does not react with the aromatic material during extraction and leaves no residue. Extraction by carbon dioxide uses very sophisticated and expensive equipment, developed to supply food grade oils to the food industry.

More recently, there is the advanced phytonics process, developed by Dr. Peter Wilde in 1987. This process is performed at cold temperatures, using possibly the cleanest technology available today. In Dr. Wilde's method, environmentally friendly, non-ozone depleting hydroflourocarbons are used to deliver a product of pharmaceutical quality.

19. What is the difference between flower essences and flower oils?

Flower essences are vibrational remedies created by placing flowers in water and exposing them to sun or moon light to extract an etheric imprint of the flower. Flower essences were developed by English doctor Edward Bach in 1930. These remedies are aimed at the etheric and electromagnetic field of the human body in order to heal illnesses of a more subtle order—emotional and mental. Precious flower oils are a physical extract of the aromatic material of the flower and can affect the mind and emotions at the same time that their therapeutic properties address conditions in the physical body.

20. Can aromatherapy interfere with homeopathic treatment?

There is no "scientifically satisfying" answer to whether aromatherapy interferes with homeopathic treatment. A vibrational medicine method, homeopathy uses a holistic system of treatment. Because this is still not easily understood by the general public, people react with extra sensitivity about it. Thought and emotion are not physical, but they can affect matter. It is generally agreed that an emotion can make the physical body sick. Can powerful emotions interfere with homeopathic treatment? Even more significant is the "thought" that the essential oils interference would affect the homeopathic treatment. French author Marguerite Maury writes about her belief in the synergy of homeopathic and aromatherapy treatments in chapter 10 of her *Guide to Aromatherapy*.

My thought on this is that if both treatments are intentionally used at once, for greatest benefit the doctor prescribing homeopathy should also be knowledgeable of aromatherapy, in order to prescribe both alternatives to work together.

Say someone is under homeopathic treatment and is having an aromatherapy massage. What happens is going to depend in large on the influence of this person's beliefs and emotions about using both therapies. If the homeopathy treatment is for an illness that is causing the individual a lot of emotional stress, it is logical to conclude that if essential oils are also being used to sedate the nervous system, it is not going against the intention and action of the homeopathic treatment, but is enhancing its action.

21. Are there different types of aromatherapy practice?

Aromatherapy is naturally divided into three distinct fields: medicinal use, cosmetic use, and use in psychology or psychotherapy.

The medical branch of aromatherapy involves an in-depth study of how the properties of each oil can affect organs and internal tissue to heal or promote healing. Oils can be taken internally under the close direction of an expert—certain oils can be toxic and must be used with experienced precision. Oils in dilution are applied on the body through the skin by massage to address certain internal conditions of the neuro-muscular system, and used externally in the treatment and prevention of bacterial or fungal infections on the skin. Oils can be introduced into the body to address conditions of the internal organs using gelatin capsules or suppositories.

France and England are at the forefront of this work; in these countries, a number of medical doctors are using aromatherapy in hospitals. In France, aromatherapy is offered in pharmaceutical and medical school.

The cosmetic branch of aromatherapy practice is in the hands of estheticians and massage therapists who use essential oils in skin care, hair, and other beauty treatments, and in relaxation therapies.

In Psycho-aromatherapy, the use of essential oils is applied to psychotherapy. This involves the study of the relationship between memory and emotion and scent, and how that can be used to improve the individual's emotional or mental condition. It can be called "therapy by aroma."

22. Can you say a word on the toxicity of essential oils?

The first thing to remember is that because essential oils are natural, botanical substances, this does not guarantee safety. Fortunately, the most poisonous plants are not aromatic and the majority of essential oils (85 to 90 percent) are quite safe to use.

The next thing to consider is quantity and concentration, meaning how much essential oil is diluted in a vegetable oil, for example, to be used either internally or externally.

Essential oils are 70 times more concentrated than the plant that they were extracted from. Ingestion of essential oils should only be done under precise instruction for dosage. Care should be taken also in the dilution of oils for external use, and in the frequency of application.

Robert Tisserand studied this subject extensively and, in *The Essential Oil Safety Data Manual,* he classifies essential oils hazards into three categories:

Toxicity: different degrees of poisoning.

Irritation: inflammation of mucus membranes or the skin. (Frequency of application in relation to the body's response to irritation is important here.)

Sensitation: allergic reaction, mostly manifesting on the skin and involving the immune system. (This can occur with small amounts and few or single applications.)

Again, remember that the majority of oils are perfectly harmless and poisoning has only been reported in cases of excessive overdose—such as 50 to 200 times above a safe dose of a toxic oil.

Since ingestion of essential oils has marked quite a long path in history—in the form of spices with toxic aromatic material—common sense concludes that the therapeutic use of essential oils will not give rise to unexpected side effects like those we risk in the case of comparably new, briefly tested synthetic chemicals.

23. Why are toxic oils produced and what are the most toxic oils?

Some toxic oils are very powerful agents to be used therapeutically. For example, an oil that can be an irritant to a certain organ can also be used to treat that organ. The positive efficiency of such therapy involves knowledge of how to apply this toxic oil in the right concentrations. It has been documented that low concentrations are very effective.

Below are listed some of the most common toxic oils in order of hazardous effects.

Toxicity: mustard, rue, savin, horseradish, pennyroyal, mugwort, hyssop, wormwood, wintergreen, thyme, fennel.

Skin sensitivity: bergamot, clove, cinnamon, cumin, pine, oregano, sassafras, savory, juniper. (Juniper berry oil is not toxic, only the juniper leaves and twigs are.)

24. Why is aromatherapy important in skin care?

The life-giving support and cell regeneration capabilities of essential oils make their utility in skin care remarkable.

Essential oils have an antiseptic effect acting against bacteria. Their amazing ability to penetrate creates an obvious advantage in skin care, not only to balance different skin conditions and treat acne, but also serving as a natural preservative in cosmetics. Since some essential oils have compounds that can be compared to hormones, they have the ability to stimulate or calm our own hormones, serving to regulate functions of the skin.

25. Can acne be cured with essential oils?

Acne is more than skin deep. Stress and diet are major factors in creating the imbalances that promote acne. It is important to mention here, however, that the aromatic experience of essential oils also has an added factor in reducing stress by relaxing the mind and body.

Certain oils have properties that can improve the skin circulation, which is usually poor in skin with acne. In addition, an oil that is a strong bactericidal, such as lemon, can help skin with acne diminish the production of bacteria and neutralize the waste products caused by it (see chapter 4).

26. Why is scent and the sense of smell associated with memory and emotion?

There has been fairly extensive research done in Europe, Japan, the United States, and Russia on the subject of the association of memory, emotion, and the sense of smell. Internal nasal membranes contain the olfactory receptors, but the olfactory bulb is inside the cranial area. Our sense of smell is processed in the brain, below the hypothalamus, in the cortex. This is the same area of the brain where memory and emotion are processed. This part of our brain is the most primitive, an area that was present in the development of the lower evolution—nicknamed "the smell brain"—the rhinecephalon.

In primitive man, as well as in modern man, information needed from memory and emotion strongly depends on the sense of smell to trigger action and behavior regarding the gathering of food, hunting, migration, escape, sexual inter-action, and the processing of more subtle information.

27. How do memory, emotion, and scent association relate to aromatherapy?

Presently, there are a small number of psycho-aromathera-pists, myself included, who are using essential oils with the memory/emotion and scent association as a tool to apply different methods of therapy to heal the emotional and mental condition of patients. This practice is of great use in psychotherapy, especially in shock conditions, for hospital patients and for substance addiction patients in rehabilita-tion centers.

28. How and when was the word aromatherapy first used?

The term *aromatherapy* was first coined by French chemist René-Maurice Gattefossé who, by accident, rediscovered the therapeutic properties of essential oils. In 1928, Gattefossé was working in his family's perfumery lab when he got a severe burn on his hand while handling some of the lab equipment. The botanical oil of lavender was used as a wash after the accident. Following this incident, he noticed that the lavender oil had stopped the spread of gangrenous sores that were developing on his tissue. The burn healed rapidly and with little scarring. He became fascinated by this fact and began researching the antiseptic and antibiotic properties of essential oils. Later his studies attracted interest in France, Germany, and Switzerland, thus gathering a small group in the scientific community in Europe, among whom are Dr. Jean Valnet, Dr. Jean Claude Lapraz, Dr. Daniel Pénoël, and research scientist Pierre Franchomme, who continues to work with medical aromatherapy.

Forty years later, Robert Tisserand succeeded in spreading the word *aromatherapy* in Europe and the United States by publishing his popular book *The Art of Aromatherapy*.

29. What is the future of aromatherapy?

As most societal accomplishments often begin with one individual, it is easy to observe that the natural path aromatherapy is taking began with the rediscovery and growth in knowledge from Gattefossé, reached a group of serious researchers, and now it is taking ground in the societies of the world in many forms.

Environmental fragrancing, a term already in current use in many countries, seems to be one of the important avenues of action affecting society, which is going to teach us about the power of the aromatic experience in many areas of our lives, all over the world. Avid research and current applications active now in Japan use the therapeutic properties of essential oils in the workplace, using modern techniques of diffusing aromatic molecules in office buildings and in the home. In England, the essential oil of lavender is used as a deodorizer in the subway transportation system. In France, doctors have found that the dispersion of essential oils in hospitals helps to control the proliferation of airborne germs and viruses.

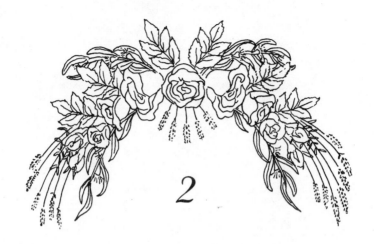

2

The Essential Oils

The Apprentice's List

$\mathcal{T}$he list of essential oils in this chapter contains the most important oils for the beginner to learn to use and the oils most immediately available through most stores selling essential oils.

My source of information for writing this chapter relied on the works of Dr. Kurt Schnaubelt, Dr. Pénoël, Pierre Franchomme, Robert Tisserand, Julia Lawless, Dr. Jean Valnet, and others. For further study and reputable essential oils labels for aromatherapy, refer to the appendix.

All essential oils lend themselves to a wide variety of actions that describe their properties. This chapter lists only the most prominent actions for each oil described for the purpose of quick reference. See the descriptions of these properties at the end of this chapter for further information.

Below is a list of the oils included in this chapter:

Basil *(Ocimum basilicum)*
Bergamot *(Citrus bergamia)*
Chamomile *(Chamaemelum nobile* and
   Matricaria recutica)
Eucalyptus *(Eucalyptus globulus)*
Frankincense *(Boswellia carterii)*
Geranium *(Pelargonium graveolens)*
Jasmine *(Jasminum officinale)*
Lavender *(Lavendula angustifolia)*
Lemon *(Citrus limon)*
Mint, peppermint *(Mentha piperita)*
Orange Blossom (Neroli) *(Citrus aurantium)*
Rose *(Rosa damascena)*
Rosemary *(Rosmarinus officinalis)*
Sage, clary *(Salvia sclarea)*
Sandalwood *(Santalum album)*
Tea Tree *(Melaleuca alternifolia)*
Ylang Ylang *(Cananga odorata)*

Basil

Ocimum basilicum

Botanical family: Labiatae.

Principle components: Linalol, eugenol, limonene.

Climate of origin: Tropical. Native to Asia and Africa.

Oil extracted from: Herb; leaves and flowers.

Produced in: Egypt, France, India, Pacific Islands, United States, and Brazil.

Blending class: Top note.

Characteristics: Yellow oil, fresh, herbacious "green" odor, bittersweet taste. Blends well with clary sage, geranium, lavender, lime. Used in perfumery and the food industry.

History and lore: Used widely in India's Ayurvedic medicine known as *tulsi*. Used to treat bronchitis, coughs, flu, and stomach ailments. Also used as an antidote against snake and venomous insect bites, taken internally or applied on the skin.

Basil has been associated with the scorpion, the planet Mars, and the element fire.

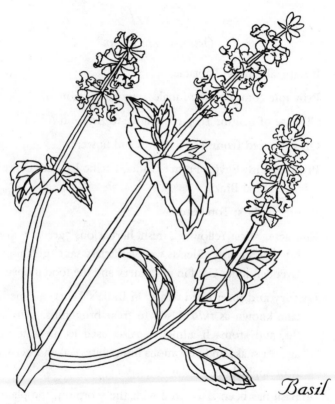

Basil

Ocimum basilicum

Therapeutic properties: Relieves smooth muscle spasms, indicated for nausea; stimulant for the mind in depressive states; insect repellent and mosquito bite relief. Think of basil when you feel that kind of nervousness that affects your stomach and gives you pangs and nausea; also think of basil when your mind feels gray and slow and your mental focus is failing you, leading to depressive states. Avoid in the first trimester of pregnancy.

Actions: Antispasmodic, cephalic, stimulant, antidepressant.

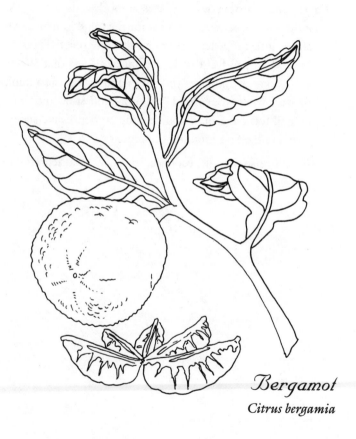

Bergamot

Citrus bergamia

Bergamot
Citrus bergamia

Botanical family: Rutaceae.

Principle components: Linalyl acetate, linalol, sesquiter-pines bergapten.

Climate of origin: Tropical; native to Asia.

Oil extracted from: Rind of fruit.

Produced in: Italy and the Ivory Coast.

Blending class: Top note.

Characteristics: Light green oil with a fresh sweet scent. Blends well with all citrus and flower oils including lavender, geranium, and juniper.

History and lore: Bergamot oil has been widely used in Italian folk medicine. It was first sold in Italy in the town of Bergamo, from which its name is derived.

One of its components, a furocoumarins called bergapten, has been found to cause skin pigmentation—staining skin if exposed to sunlight—and possible sensitization, even in dilution.

It is one of the ingredients of the classic eau de cologne and is widely used in the food and fragrance industry.

Ruled by the sun and the element fire.

Therapeutic properties: Bergamot oil has been used for treating infection on the mucous membranes of the mouth, throat, respiratory, urinary tracts, and of the female organs (used in douches and sitzs baths). It is useful as an antiseptic against infection caused by organisms such as gonococcus, staphylococcus, coli, meningococcus, and diphtheria bacillus.

Actions: Analgesic, antiseptic, cicatrisant, deodorant, and sedative.

Chamomile

Two types of chamomile are included

Roman Chamomile

Chamaemelum nobile

Botanical family: Compositae.

Principle components: Pinocarvone, farnesol, pinene, neroli-dol, cineol.

Climate of origin: Temperate to cold climates; native to southwest Europe.

Oil extracted from: Herb and flowers.

Produced in: Belgium, England, France, Hungary, and Italy.

Blending class: Top note.

Characteristics: White flowers with yellow center, yielding a pale blue liquid when new, turning yellow with age. An apple-like scent, sweet and warm, but has a bitter taste. Blends well with clary sage, geranium, jasmine, lavender, and neroli.

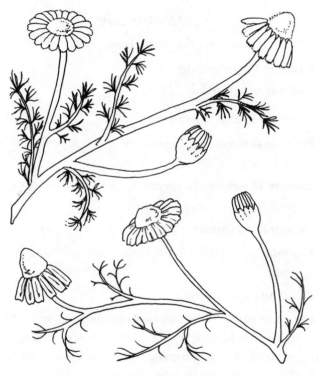

German Chamomile

Matricaria recutica

History and lore: Used by several cultures such as Egyptians, Greeks, Moors, and Anglo Saxons. Its use was widely spread throughout the Mediterranean region and was called the "plant's physician," for the popular belief that this herb kept other garden plants healthy. In the Middle Ages it was planted on the garden path so that as it was stepped on, it would release its apple-like scent.

Associated with the moon and the element water, it was one of the Saxons' nine sacred herbs.

Used in perfumery and in the food industry.

Therapeutic properties: Helpful as a sedative in nervous states having to do with physical impact such as shock, blows, and injury affecting the nervous system. Wonderful for calming infants. A good remedy for asthma with nervous origin and for intestinal parasites.

Actions: Analgesic, antispasmodic, cicatrisant, hepatic, and sedative.

German Chamomile
Matricaria recutica, blue chamomile

This chamomile contains chamazulene as its principle component, also known as azulene, a very powerful substance consisting of anti-inflammatory blue crystals. Azulene is formed as the essential oil of *matricaria recutica*, distilled from the flowers. Think of chamomile to counteract the inflamed red tissue (internally or externally) that produces swelling, bruises, rashes, rheumatic pains, sore muscles, and teething aches. German chamomile is also called "blue chamomile."

In appearance it is ink blue. An absolute is also produced from the flowers, which is a fixative with a more viscous consistency. Its odor is stronger, warmer, and sweeter than Roman chamomile.

It is native to Europe and northwest Asia. The oil is currently produced in Hungary and Germany.

Therapeutic properties: Tonic for the digestive system used to treat dyspepsia and gastro-intestinal ulcers. Also used to treat inflamed conditions on the skin such as acne and dermatosis, and internal organ tissue inflammations.

Actions: Anti-inflammatory, antispasmodic, anti-allergic, tonic, and cicatrisant.

Eucalyptus
Eucalyptus globulus

Botanical family: Myrtaceae.

Principle components: Eucalyptol, cineol, pinene, limonene, terpinene.

Climate of origin: Tropical, sub-tropical to dry temperate. Native to Australia.

Oil extracted from: Leaves.

Produced in: Spain, Portugal, Brazil, California.

Blending class: Top note; not recommended for perfumery.

Characteristics: White to yellow liquid with somewhat harsh, strong odor; mild bitter taste; blends well with lavender, rosemary, lemon. Used extensively in the pharmaceutical industry for a wide variety of medical preparations, and as a flavoring agent in the food industry.

History and lore: Used in Australia for respiratory problems and, secondarily, on the skin for burns and wounds. The leaves are smoked for asthma and applied on open wounds for fast healing. Ruled by the planet Saturn and the element Earth.

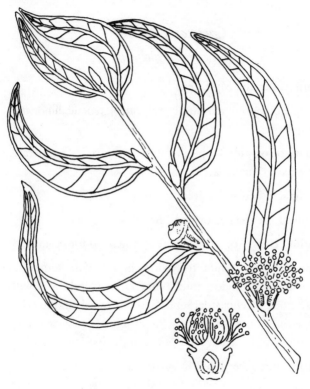

Eucalyptus

Eucalyptus globulus

Therapeutic properties: The eucalyptus oil can be used in massage blends to relieve muscular aches and joint pain, and to improve poor circulation.

Eucalyptus is a remedy for outbreaks of herpes simplex (lip sores). It can be applied neat to reduce the virus cycle time for closing and to relieve the pain. In cases of bronchitis, it is used in inhalations or applied diluted in massage on the lung area (back of chest).

Actions: Analgesic, anti-viral, expectorant, stimulant.

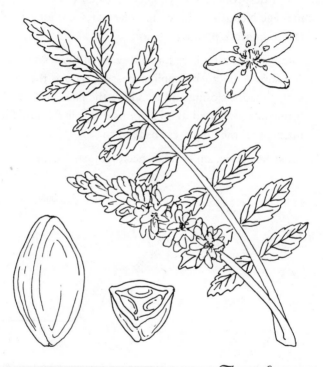

Frankincense

Boswellia carterii

Frankincense
Boswellia carterii

Botanical family: Burseraceae.

Principle components: Terpinene, pinene, dipentene, limonene, thujene, cymene, incensole, octylacetate.

Climate of origin: Sub-tropical dry climates. Native to the Red Sea region.

Oil extracted from: Gum resin from small tree.

Produced in: South Arabia, Somalia, Ethiopia, China.

Blending class: Base note.

Characteristics: Clear to yellow liquid with a woody/spicy odor. Used in the pharmaceutic and perfume industries, in the manufacture of incense, and to a smaller degree in the food industry as a flavoring agent.

History and lore: Frankincense was highly regarded in the ancient civilizations of the Middle East and Africa. One of the gifts of the wise men to the infant Christ, it was considered as valuable as gold. Commerce negotiations for frankincense were esteemed as primary importance.

The Egyptians used frankincense for their famous rejuvenating facial masks.

In the Middle Ages, frankincense was used in hospitals to fumigate or "smoke" patients suffering from evil spirits (madness).

In India, it was used for treatment of all kinds of internal and external infections. Frankincense is ruled by the Sun and the element fire.

Therapeutic properties: Treatment of infected wounds, it is a strong astringent useful in inhalations for catarral conditions of the lungs. Also used to draw out genitourinary tract infections.

In skin care, frankincense is used for mature skin and wrinkle formulas.

Soothing effect on the mind and emotions.

Actions: Antiseptic, astringent, cicatrisant, sedative.

Geranium

Pelargonium graveolens

Botanical family: Geraniaceae.

Principle components: Geraniol, citronellol, linalol, and limonene.

Climate of origin: Sub-tropical. Native to South Africa.

Oil extracted from: The whole plant with flowers.

Produced in: China and Madagascar.

Blending class: Middle note.

Characteristics: Green liquid with strong sweet/fresh odor and bitter taste. Blends well with any oil, especially with lavender, rose, sandalwood, basil, and all citrus oils.

Used in the fragrance and food industry.

History and lore: Since antiquity, geranium has been well regarded for treating all female complaints, such as excessive menstruation, hot flashes, and vaginitis. Ruled by the planet Venus and the element Earth.

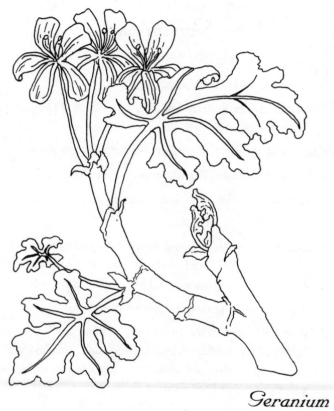

Geranium

Pelargonium graveolens

Therapeutic properties: Geranium is a stimulant of the adrenal cortex, where sex hormones are produced. It is believed that geranium can act as a balancing stimulant for female organs and the nervous system. It can be applied on sores such as vaginal herpes and other inflamed conditions of the vaginal mucous membranes to relieve pain. It is used for eczema treatments and as an insect repellent. As an analgesic/astringent it is also helpful in breast engorgement and hemorrhoids.

Actions: Analgesic, antiseptic, astringent, cicatrisant, and hemostatic.

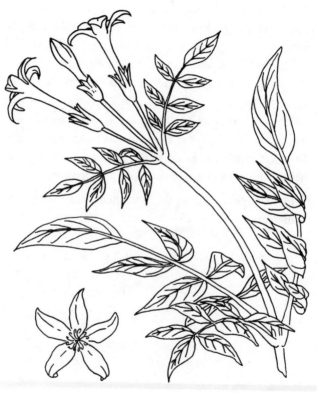

Jasmine

Jasminum officinale

Jasmine
Jasminum officinale

Botanical family: Jasminaceae.

Principle components: Benzyl acetate, benzyl alcohol, cis-jasmone, linalol, farnesol, indole, methy jasmonate.

Climate of origin: Native to China and Asia.

Oil extracted from: Flower.

Produced in: India, France, Morocco, Egypt, Japan, China, and Italy.

Blending class: Base note.

Characteristics: Reddish brown viscous liquid with an inebriating sweet floral scent; blends well with most essences.

History and lore: Jasmine has long been a favorite of Eastern nations and has an established reputation as an aphrodisiac and indispensable ingredient in sensual massage to relax the body. In China, jasmine flowers are used to scent tea. Jasmine flowers must be picked at night during their yearly season. In India, jasmine is nicknamed "moonlight of the grove." It is one of the most expensive botanical oils and is used in high class perfumery.

Ruled by the planet Jupiter and the element fire.

Therapeutic properties: Jasmine has a relaxing effect on the nervous system and has been reported to increase alpha brain waves.

In the West, jasmine has been used as a tonic to the male and female reproductive organs, as a before and after birth essence, to ease labor pains, to remedy afterbirth depression, and to help with the flow of milk.

Jasmine seems to have a marked presence in modifying depressive states of mind and in stimulating positive emotions.

Actions: Antidepressant, antispasmodic, aphrodisiac, galactogogue, and sedative.

Lavender
Lavandula officinalis

There are many varieties of the genus *lavendula,* cultivated all over the world. *Lavandula officinalis* is the general term to describe the genus. The most known varieties, *Lavandula angustifolia* or *Lavendula vera,* and *Lavandula latifolia,* by bee pollination create the hybrid lavander known as *lavandin.* All of these lavenders are different "chemotypes," meaning that their natural chemistries vary in composition and, therefore, they also vary slightly in therapeutic properties. However, all have a sedating effect on the central nervous system and can be used for antiseptic and deodorant actions.

Botanical family: Labiatae.

Principle components: Linalol, lavandulyl acetate, linalyl acetate, lavandulol, cineol, limonene, terpineol.

Climate of origin: Temperate, dry. Lavender is native to the Mediterranean region.

Oil extracted from: Herb; flowering tops.

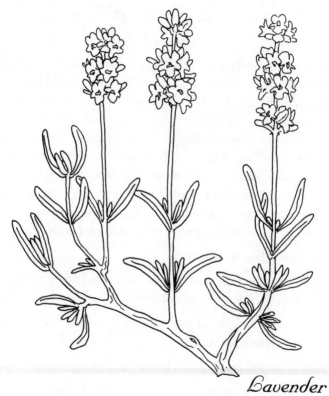

Lavender

Lavandula officinalis

Produced in: A variety of climates, temperate to cold. France, Spain, Italy, England, Australia, Greece, and Russia. The best oil comes from the French alps.

Blending class: Top note.

Characteristics: Clear liquid by steam distillation with a powerful herbal/floral odor with mild bitter taste. An absolute is also produced by solvent extraction, which produces a thicker deep green oil with a sweeter odor. Lavender blends well with most floral, citrus, and herbal oils. Widely used in the perfume industry.

History and lore: Lavender was first established in the Western world by the Romans, who used lavender extensively in their bathing rituals. The word *lavender* is derived from the Latin word *lavare*, meaning "to wash."

Lavender has a long standing tradition in the preparation of sachets, scenting linens, and in floral waters. In birthing and convalescent rooms, lavender flowers were burned to create an aura of cleanliness and to please deities.

Lavender is ruled by the planet Mercury and the element air.

Therapeutic properties: Lavender is nicknamed "the universal oil" because it lends itself to so many different uses. It is wonderful as an anti-stress agent in a bath to relax body, mind, and emotion. It is a remedy for migraines, insomnia, and nervous depression.

Lavender is a strong, non-toxic antiseptic that can be applied neat on cuts and burns to prevent infection and helps to promote fast formation of scar tissue to close a wound and can be used to treat anal fistula. A mild sedative, lavender soothes skin suffering from overexposure to the sun, mosquito and spider bite relief and repellent. In childbirth, lavender is very helpful to relax mother during contractions. It is a mild sedative in an infant's massage oil to relax the neuromuscular system after birth.

Actions: Analgesic, antiseptic, antitoxic, cicatrisant, and sedative.

Lemon

Citrus limon

Botanical family: Rutaceae.

Principle components: Limonene, linalol, pinene, geraniol, citral, terpinene, citronellal.

Climate of origin: Temperate. Native to Asia.

Oil extracted from: The rind of the fresh lemon peel.

Produced in: Spain, Portugal, Italy, Brazil, California.

Blending class: Top note.

Characteristics: A greenish yellow liquid with mild and refreshing citrus notes and a sharp, tart taste. Blends well with geranium, lavender, eucalyptus, neroli, rose, and sandalwood.

It is used extensively by the fragrance, pharmaceutical, and food industries.

History and lore: In European latin countries and South America, a household does not function without lemons. The juice of the lemon is used as a bactericide,

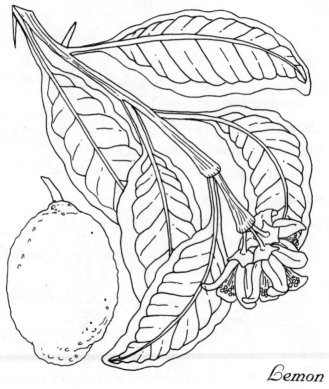

Lemon

Citrus limon

to soak and wash meat prior to cooking, and as a drink to treat infectious diseases and to reduce fever.

Therapeutic properties: The essential oil of lemon is the most powerful antiseptic of all essences. It is a good inhalation remedy for respiratory tract infections during a cold or flu.

Lemon has a tonic and detoxifying effect on the gastric mucus membranes; it promotes a healthy flow of urine and stimulates the production of white blood cells. It is thinning to the blood, and therefore helpful to those suffering from high blood pressure.

Lemon also has a neutralizing action on the liver and helps those who are anemic with liver malfunction.

Actions: Antiseptic, antitoxic, bactericidal, diuretic, febrifuge, hemostatic, hypotensive, and anti-anemic.

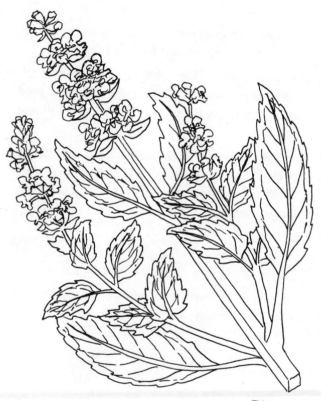

Peppermint

Mentha piperita

Mint, Peppermint
Mentha piperita

Botanical family: Labitae.

Principle components: Menthol, limonene, cineol, and menthyl acetate.

Climate of origin: The peppermint that is cultivated now is a hybrid of other mints developed in England. It is possibly original to the Mediterranean region.

Oil extracted from: Herb; the flowering plant.

Produced in: All over the world, most importantly in England, France, the United States, and China.

Blending class: Top note.

Characteristics: A light green or yellow liquid with a powerfully penetrating, zesty, camphor-like odor. It blends well with lemon, eucalyptus, lavender, and rosemary.

Used by the pharmaceutical, food, and fragrance industries.

History and lore: There is record of peppermint tracing as far back as being cultivated by the Egyptians. In Greek mythology, there is the mention of a sensual nymph called Mentha, who became dear to the god Pluto. Pluto transformed her into the herb peppermint after the displays of jealousy by his wife, the goddess Persephone.

Ruled by the planet Mercury and the element air.

Therapeutic properties: Principal aromatherapy remedy for flatulence, indigestion, and colic.

Useful to the respiratory system in the form of inhalations to relieve asthma, bronchitis, head colds, and dry coughs. Peppermint can be diluted into a massage oil to be applied locally to lungs (back of chest). Good for fainting spells and mental fatigue.

Actions: Antispasmodic, analgesic, carminative, expectorant, vasoconstrictor, cephalic.

Orange Blossom (Neroli)
Citrus aurantium

Botanical family: Rutaceae.

Principle components: Linalol, linalyl acetate, limonene, nerolidol, nerol, indole, pinene, citral, jasmine, geraniol.

Climate of origin: Temperate. Native to China and grows well in dry soil such as that in the Mediterranean region.

Oil extracted from: Flowers of the bitter orange tree.

Produced in: France, Tunisia, Italy, Morocco.

Blending class: Top note.

Characteristics: The absolute, by solvent extraction, is a reddish brown, viscous liquid with a wonderfully sweet "high pitch," mildly narcotic scent, and a bitter taste. Blends well with all essences, especially floral and citrus oils. The steam-distilled oil is light yellow in color, and is known mostly as neroli. This is a very expensive oil used in high perfumery.

History and lore: Used in China since antiquity for scenting cosmetics. Traditionally, a favorite of many countries

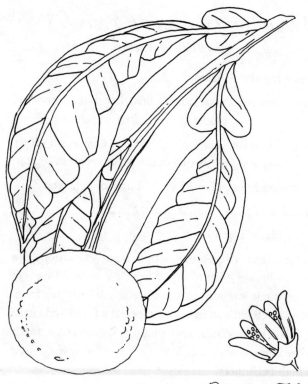

Orange Blossom
Citrus aurantium

for bridal bouquets and headdresses. This custom is attributed to the fact that the pretty smell of orange flowers can sedate the bride on her wedding day. A tranquilizing tea from the leaves and flowers of the bitter orange tree would often be given to the bride prior to attending the ceremony.

The nickname "neroli" probably came from the princess of Nerola, who was the first to set the trend of perfuming leather gloves with the scent of orange blossoms.

In Arabian countries, the orange blossom water, a by-product of the flower distillation process, is used as a digestive drinking water and in the preparation of fine pastries.

Ruled by the Sun and the element fire.

Therapeutic properties: If lemon oil is the most important aromatherapy antiseptic, neroli is the most important sedative. It has an action on the heart, slowing cardiac contractions in palpitations and spasms. It is of great value in therapies dealing with sudden shock or unbearable stress, as in cases of hysteria, anxiety, fear of death, grief, and strong emotions affecting the heart. It can be used in cases of nervous diarrhea, and helps to eliminate intestinal gas and colic. A relaxing bath can be made to treat nervous depression.

Neroli is non-toxic. The orange blossom water is an excellent soothing drink for infants' colic and for insomnia.

Actions: Antidepressant, aphrodisiac, cordial, digestive.

Rose

Two types of rose are included

Among the more than 10,000 varieties of rose, there are three distinct varieties cultivated for rose oil production: *Rosa centifolia, Rosa gallica,* and *Rosa damascena.*

The rose known as *Rose maroc,* or Cabbage rose, is a hybrid combining the pink *Rosa centifolia* with the red rose *Rosa gallica,* and used for the production of the true extract of rose, the "absolute."

Rosa gallica was the apothecary's garden rose, widely used by monks and alchemists in the medicinal preparations of early Europe. *Rosa damascena*, a fragile and fragrant variety, is cultivated in Bulgaria and Turkey for the production of steam distilled "otto."

Rosa centifolia

Botanical family: Rosaceae.

Principle components: Phenyl ethanol, geranial, nerol, citronellol, stearopten, farnesol, plus hundreds of others in minute traces.

Climate of origin: Temperate.

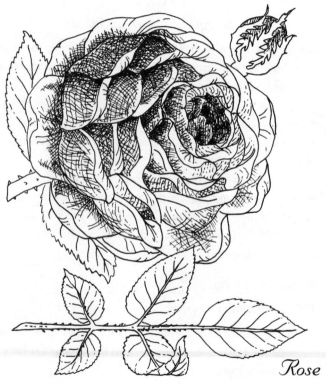

Rose

Rosa maroc

Produced in: Morocco, France, England, Italy, China.

Blending class: Base note.

Characteristics: The otto is a light yellow liquid with a warm, sweet odor. The absolute is a reddish orange denser oil with a richer sweet aroma. Blends well with most essential oils.

History and lore: Used extensively during medieval times as a "cure all" medicine and is still of prime importance in Ayurvedic and Chinese medicine. The Greeks regarded the rose as the flower of Aphrodite (Venus), Goddess of beauty and love. The most feminine of all scents, the perfume of rose has been used as an aphrodisiac and for magic rituals throughout history. Since early times, the rose essence has been known to have a therapeutic action to the heart and womb by regulating excessive bleeding.

Ruled by Venus and the element Earth.

Therapeutic properties: Rose oil can be used for balancing female sexual organ disorders, hemorrhages, mastitis, stress-related problems, impotence, frigidity, irritable and sensitive skin, eczema, broken capillaries, poor circulation, headaches, hay fever, and liver disorders.

Actions: Aphrodisiac, uterine, sedative, astringent, rubefacient, hemostatic, hepatic.

Rosa damascena

Botanical family: Rosaceae.

Principle components: Citronellol, geraniol, stearopten, nerol, phenyl ethanol, farnesol, and many others.

Climate of origin: Temperate; native to the Far East.

Produced in: Bulgaria, France, and Turkey.

Blending class: Base note.

Characteristics: A light yellow, sometimes faintly green liquid that can solidify at room temperature. It has a tart/sweet narcotic-like scent, very powerful and is not commonly pleasant to the unaccustomed person in its undiluted form. One drop or less of this otto can go a long way in a blend. Bulgarian rose otto is one of the most expensive essential oils. It takes from 30 to 60 roses to produce a single drop of rose oil. Used in high perfumery.

Note that in India, a perfume called "aytar"—a combination of rose and sandalwood—became famous all over the world. Do not confuse this with the name "otto," which refers to the pure steam-distilled rose oil.

History and lore: This cultivated rose may have been developed in Persia in ancient times. Legend tells of a princess' wedding for which the garden was cut with canals. For the ceremony, roses were placed on the water of these canals. With the heat, rose essence appeared floating visibly on the surface of the water. Supposedly, after this incident, the Persians were the first to develop a distillation process to obtain the rose oil. This rose is now cultivated in Morocco, France, Italy, and China.

For properties and actions see *Rosa centifolia*.

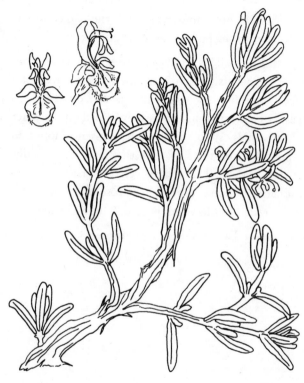

Rosemary

Rosmarinus officinalis

Rosemary
Rosmarinus officinalis

Botanical family: Labiatae.

Principle components: Pinene, limonene, linalol, cineol, borneol, camphene, terpineol.

Climate of origin: Temperate dry, desert; native to the mediterranean region.

Oil extracted from: Herb; the whole plant with flowering tops.

Produced in: France, Tunisia, Morocco, Spain, China.

Blending class: Middle note.

Characteristics: Clear liquid with a penetrating green fresh/herbal scent; relatively mellow minty taste; blends well with basil, peppermint, lemon, lavender.

History and lore: The influence of the piercing scent of rosemary has been recognized since early times in European medicine as a remedy for "weakness of the brain." In France, fumigations (burning to cause an aromatic smoke; smudging) were prepared in hospitals to get rid of "evil spirits."

Rosemary tea was used to awaken the senses and liven the memory.

Rosemary facial wash was used as a beautifying agent, tinctures of it were used to darken the hair, and this herb was often present in culinary uses for flavoring meats and other dishes.

The mere presence of this plant was believed to drive away fever. Used extensively in medieval magic rituals. In ancient Greece, it was regarded as a sacred herb.

Ruled by the Sun and the element fire.

Therapeutic properties: Activates lethargic circulation during respiratory infections. Clears nasal passages during colds, bronchitis, and whooping cough.

Rosemary can be used in massage for rheumatism, gout, varicose veins, and any condition due to poor circulation. Stimulates the scalp and helps reconstruct the damaged hair follicle. Rosemary is also useful for the digestive system as it serves as a remedy for colitis and flatulence. Avoid in the first trimester of pregnancy.

Actions: Antispasmodic, carminative, cephalic, decongestant, digestive, stimulant, sudorific.

Sage, Clary
Salvia sclarea

Botanical family: Labiatae.

Principle components: Linalyl acetate, linalol, pinene, myrcene.

Climate of origin: Temperate dry, desert. Native to the Middle East and south of Europe.

Oil extracted from: Herb; flowering top and leaves.

Produced in: Bulgaria, France, Morocco, and Spain

Blending class: Middle note.

Characteristics: A light greenish yellow liquid with a pleasant herbal scent and mild bitter taste. Blends well with other herbal and citrus oils, but also with woods such as cedarwood and sandalwood.

History and lore: This herb was well liked by medieval herbalists and healers. The mucilaginous seeds were used for making a soothing, slippery tea to wash and "clear" foreign bodies from the eyes. The denomination clary is thought of as coming from this use of the herb. Clary sage

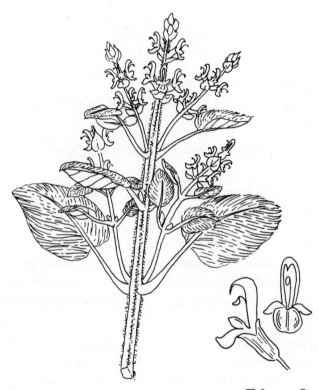

Clary Sage

Salvia sclarea

has been known to have a narcotic-like effect, as documented by Robert Tisserand in *The Art of Aromatherapy*.

Used widely in the fragrance and food industry.

Ruled by Mercury and the element air.

Therapeutic properties: Clary sage is both sedative and tonic, so think of clary when the condition is one of weakness coming from the nervous system and causing general physical debility or apathy. Good for use in any convalescent state. Clary sage has been used as a panacea since ancient times. Its high content of the aromatic component linalol qualifies it as an anesthetic.

I have massaged diluted clary on the lower abdomen to successfully diminish menstrual cramps. It has a wonderful nurturing and soothing quality. Clary sage is a good companion for harmonization of the female cycle, but you must avoid in the first trimester of pregnancy.

Actions: Antidepressant, antispasmodic, anesthetic, hypotensor, sedative, tonic.

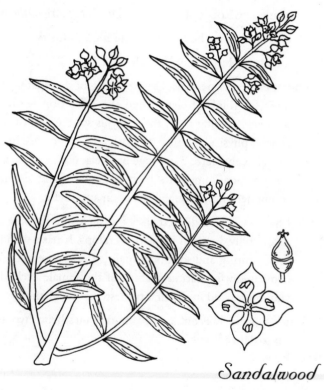

Sandalwood

Santalum album

Sandalwood
Santalum album

Botanical family: Santalaceae.

Principle components: Santalol, borneol, santalone, santine and other trace sesquiterpine hydrocarbons.

Climate of origin: Tropical; native to Asia.

Oil extracted from: Wood; the inner "heart" wood.

Produced in: India (Mysore), Indonesia, and Taiwan.

Blending class: Base note.

Characteristics: A heavy viscous clear to yellow oil with a wonderful sweet wood scent and a bitter hot taste.

Blends well with most essential oils and herbs, as well as with resin and all floral oils.

History and lore: Sandalwood has been used for at least 4,000 years, and is often associated with meditation temples of the East. In India it is combined with rose oil to produce the famous perfume aytar. In Asia, the wood is used in the wood carvings of scented boxes, furniture, and fine building. Sandalwood is an incense, a main ingredient in the production of cosmetics and for embalming. It is also used as a moisturizer for dry and rough skin.

Used by the fragrance industry as a fixative in high perfumery and cosmetics.

Ruled by Uranus and the element air.

Therapeutic properties: In Ayurvedic medicine, sandalwood is used for treating urinary, respiratory infections, and diarrhea. In Chinese medicine, it is a remedy for choleric intestines, stomach conditions, vomiting, and gonorrhea.

Currently, sandalwood is used in English hospitals for the treatment of streptococcus throat infections.

Actions: Antiseptic, aphrodisiac, bactericidal, anti-phlogistic, expectorant, sedative.

Tea Tree
Melaleuca alternifolia

Botanical family: Myrtaceae.

Principle components: Terpinene-4-ol, sesquiterpenes, cineol, pinene.

Climate of origin: Sub-tropical. Native to Australia.

Oil extracted from: Leaves and twigs.

Produced in: Australia.

Blending class: Middle note.

Characteristics: Light yellow or greenish oil with a very strong, balsamic/spicy, medicinal smell. It can yield a fresh note when blended with geranium, lavender, or pine.

History and lore: Tea tree has been used in Australia for a long time, originally by the aboriginal Indians. The name is attributed to the use of the leaves of this tree for a medicinal tea.

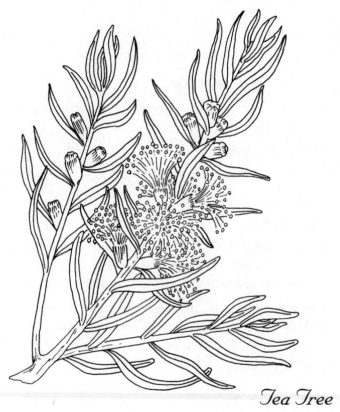

Tea Tree

Melaleuca alternifolia

Therapeutic properties: Tea tree has a peculiar property, which is to combine anti-bacterial, anti-fungal, and anti-viral actions, thus serving as if it were many oils combined. Its most important therapeutic power is the stimulation of the immunological system.

Tea tree is a general antiseptic and cicatrisant and it is non-toxic. It can be used in any condition needing an anti-infectious action.

Actions: Antiseptic, anti-bactericide, anti-viral, anti-fungal, immunostimulant, cicatrisant, and expectorant.

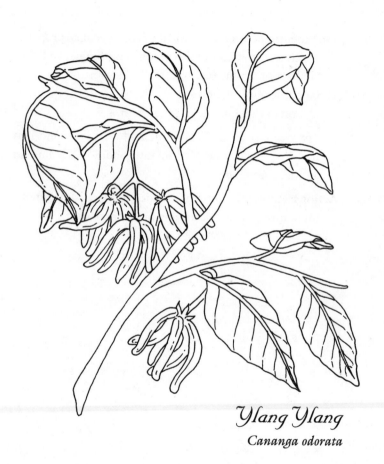

Ylang Ylang
Cananga odorata

Ylang Ylang
Cananga odorata

Botanical family: Anonaceae.

Principle components: Linalol, farnesol, benzyl acetate, methyl para-cretol.

Climate of origin: Tropical. Native to Asia.

Oil extracted from: Flowers.

Produced in: Madagascar, Comoro Islands.

Blending class: Base note.

Characteristics: Yellow in color, its scent is rather deep and strongly sweet. Serves well as a fixative in perfumery. Oil is produced with same flowers being distilled in successive distillations. First, or extra; second; third; and complete, which is a mixture of all consecutive distillations.

History and lore: Widely used in perfumery as a floral oriental note. It was used in Victorian Europe as a hair preparation. In Indonesia, where it grows, it is a tradition to cover a newly wedded couple's bed with these fragrant flowers. Oil is produced in different qualities.

Therapeutic properties: An excellent medicine for stress-related conditions, ylang ylang is a sexual tonic helpful in frigidity and impotence.

Actions: Anti-spasmodic, sexual stimulant, sedative.

Definitions of Therapeutic Actions

Analgesic: Eliminates pain.

Antidepressant: Uplifts negative states of mind.

Antiphlogistic: Constricts capillaries leading to reduction of inflammation.

Antiseptic: Substance that acts against the growth of bacteria. Antispasmodic. Relieves smooth muscle spasms.

Antispasmodic: Relaxes muscles suffering involuntary contractions.

Antitoxic: A substance acting against poisoning.

Aphrodisiac: Stimulates libido.

Astringent: A substance that contracts tissues.

Carminative: Expels gas from intestines.

Cephalic: Relates to mental disorders, stimulates memory, and sharpens focus.

Cicatrisant: Helps in the formation of scar tissue.

Cordial: Gives energy to the cardiac muscle and tones it.

Digestive: Promotes easy digestion.

Expectorant: Expels mucus from lungs, throat, and sinus.

Galactagogue: Stimulates lactation.

Hemostatic: Stops bleeding, helps blood coagulation.

Hepatic: Invigorates the liver and tones it.

Hypotensor: Lowers arterial blood pressure.

Rubefacient: Local stimulant of circulation, causing redness of skin.

Sedative: Calming action to the nervous system.

Stimulant: Speeds up metabolism.

Sudorific: Promotes or increases perspiration.

Tonic: Gives energy; invigorates the body, an organ, or local tissue.

Uterine: Tonic to the uterus.

Vasoconstrictor: Constricts capillaries.

Vulnerary: Aids in healing external wounds.

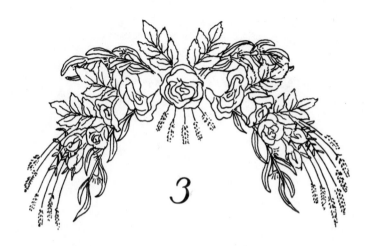

3

Blending Essential Oils

Botanical Perfume Making

The Egyptians related to perfume as a life-giving substance, and so deeply were they taken by the power of aromatic plants that one of their creation myths depicts an aromatic blue lotus flower as the first manifested form from which their God Ra, the Sun, emerged. The Egyptians perfected techniques for extracting aromatic material from plants for use in cosmetics, medicine, and spiritual practices that used incense and perfumes.

Evidence from Memphis hieroglyphs tells us of the god of perfume, Nefertum, who was associated with the aromatic lotus of creation. Nefertum, as the soul of life, would purify the body. (S. Van Toller and G. Dodd, eds. *Fragrance: The Psychology and Biology of Perfume*. New York: Elsevier Applied Science Publications, 1992, p. 290.)

In modern times, we are so bombarded with sophisticated synthetic aroma chemicals that the confusion of our olfactory system often does not permit appreciation of pure blends containing oils from plants and flowers. As a civilization, how far do we now find ourselves from the Egyptian way of honoring the Earth!

True botanical oils have a different "signature"; they are much more vibrant and earthy in spite of their more gentle interaction with the body. Modern perfumes all use synthetic fixers—substances to keep aromatic molecules from evaporating quickly from the skin. Botanical perfumes interact with the skin, then naturally disappear into the environment as if to remind us that their movement connects us to what lies beyond the physical world.

To a nose trained in botanical essential oils, what is the aromatic message of the commercial perfume? Very simple, no mysteries:

I am sophisticated, techno-smart, city inspired, and concrete wise. I am here to stay on your skin over sweat and showers for at least 36 hours. In your heart, I constantly hook you up to the high caste of society. In your mind, I

constantly remind you of the fashion models I am associ-
ated with, between the strips in the magazines . . . . You
can become me . . . through me, you will be like a million
other identity seekers, unwavering believers . . . . Little
do you know how I can hide your true identity. I can res-
cue you from human odor and give you a sexy cross
between a bon-bon and a space shuttle lubricant with a
few faux flowers sprinkled over it.

Perhaps this assessment is being a little ungrateful to the
tremendous scientific effort to lift us off the ground, but
when the mind transcends science, and modern ideas
become passe, spirit always remains.

Spirit is what I like to call the dynamics of botanical
essence—something that moves and changes like life does,
that which holds the mystery of crossing the doorway to the
invisible dimensions of existence.

I love to remember my own smell. It tells me a lot about
who I am.

When I spread a pure flower essence on my skin, I think
about that flower and her world. When the scent disappears,
does it go back to the dimension of flower consciousness?

When my own body smell merges with the scent of that flower, I am clearly aware of an interactive natural synergy.

Aromatherapists and botanical perfumers seek knowledge, knowledge about our relationship with the plant world. It is exciting to think of becoming aware of the vibrational codes coming from a plant whispering messages about life on earth.

Blending Essential Oils

When you blend essential oils, you are working with the visible oils and their physical properties and the invisible elements of their smell that will serve as your guide.

There are some common-sense facts about blending that we will begin to explore in this chapter, but there is also the level of learning about blending that relies on experience and intuition. Experience can only come with time, and in this art, it comes with smelling, blending, applying, and observing, so if you are interested in aromatherapy, you ought to start smelling essential oils as often as possible. This will naturally make memory records for the smells in your mind. Soon you will be gathering experience and feeling more and more confident in what you are doing with the oils.

Intuition is very important in blending, and I believe intuition can be invoked if the right state of mind is exercised. We all have the same potential, but this potential needs to be activated in order to function. Sometimes I think about blending in the same way I think about cooking: it's an alchemical process that involves more than what you do with your hands and a recipe to turn out great. What is in the mind matters, and the motivation and intention is principal. I tell my students that the most important intention to begin with is to create a harmonious blend by having a harmonious mind as you work, holding the feeling of believing in the abilities of the self. Choose to create something simple, and don't mix more than three oils to start. Take the three oils and learn about them first. There is so much to learn about how concentrations work in blending, even with just two oils! Safe choices for blending are oils that contain the same components. (See chapter 2.)

Oils have a character relating to their composition, the climate they grew in, the altitude at which they grew, and the soil, just to mention a few factors. Since essential oils have therapeutic properties, I find it easy to equate their character with their healing function.

Plant life assists human beings at all levels: physical, emotional, mental, and spiritual. This is an important reason to think of your blend holistically. When you are blending oils for a formula, this formula ideally should address body, mind, spirit, and emotion. In this way, your work becomes the art of putting together something synergistic, not only by the fact that the separate oils must enhance each other in the blending to create a greater sum than the separate parts combined (the concept of synergy), but that the separate therapeutic properties must also synergize to bring a total harmonization of body, mind, spirit, and emotion. Consider the holistic need of who you do aromatherapy for before you focus your intention in the search for an end result.

Next, you must know how to dilute oils in the right proportions. You will be using mostly vegetable oils as carriers for your essential oils. Essential oils don't go rancid, but vegetable oils do, so you will have to add vitamin E to your blend as a natural preservative. You can also blend essential oils into alcohol or vinegar.

Following is a list of vegetable oils you can use:

Almond oil: Sweet and fine, but I find it the most fragile oil for spoiling. Use with a few drops of vitamin E and blend small quantities at a time.

Avocado oil: Vitamin rich, highly nutritious oil, good for facial oil blends for dry and depleted skins. Fairly resistant to spoilage.

Grapeseed oil: Grapeseed is a lot like almond oil, but it has a vitamin E content that makes it more resistant to oxidation or rancidity. It is an all-purpose oil and good for massage blends.

Hazelnut oil: Fine and luxurious, with a sweet aroma.

Jojoba oil: Actually a liquid wax and not an oil. Carrier for perfume blend concentrations. Does not oxidize.

Sesame oil: Wonderful, even plain, for a sun lotion; it has a mild natural sunscreen.

I like to use the less common rice bran and aloe vera oil for its extreme fine texture in face and baby oils. It is good to blend aloe vera oil with a small amount of a more nutritious oil, such as the vegetable nut oils listed above.

About Your Blend
Concentration

Keep in mind that the concentration of essential oils inside the living plant is usually between 3 percent to 10 percent. You may create concentrate blends to be extended later, according to the application. Also, perfumes can be "extrates," a higher concentration, up to 35 percent essential oils and absolutes. I recommend beginners use low concentrations in their blends to begin, for the purpose of understanding how blends can be therapeutically powerful in low concentrations. Molecules in dispersion go through the layers of skin much more easily. Using low concentrations will also be safer and help to train the beginner's sense of smell.

The measurements given below will vary depending on the density of each oil and the drop applicator. The denser the oil, the fewer drops you will need.

1 ounce = approximately 30 ml (29.57 ml)
10% of one ounce = approximately 60 to 90 drops
1 milliliter = 20 to 35 drops
1 drop = 0.03 milliliter

Following is a list with basic guidelines on average concentrations:

Bath: 5 to 15 drops per bath, depending on oils.

Massage oil: 10 to 15 drops per ounce.

Lotion: 15 drops per ounce.

Facial oil: 6 to 12 drops per ounce.

Facial clay: 4 to 6 drops per ounce.

Hair treatment oil: 20 drops per ounce.

Fragrance: 10 percent to 35 percent concentration.

Botanical Perfume Making

When blending oils to create a perfume, think of smells as you would colors: there is no guarantee that two pretty colors will look prettier after you have mixed them. The aspect that you have to work with, besides your intuition and experience, is to learn about chemical compatibility. (For component listings see chapter 2.) Odor intensity is important because one oil can completely overpower another. Take pieces of blotter or watercolor paper and pour one drop of each oil you want to blend, separately. Notice and maybe even determine how long it takes for each smell to go away. This will give you a pretty good idea of odor intensity. The most persistent scent should be used a lot less in your blend then the ones that are mild smelling and disappear faster. Also important is the classification of oils for blending, which is usually referred as base, middle, or top notes.

Base notes: The wise old folks who are calmer, slower, and most times physically denser. Think of them as the hard drive of a computer that has memory to store outside information. They are the fixers of botanical perfumery, they are less volatile and can keep other oils in the blend from evaporating too quickly.

Middle notes: These are the oils in a blend that can be used more generously because they are the mildest smells, the ones that "round the corners," meaning that they help equalize oppositions. They are smell mediators, acting as the diplomats of a composition, negotiating chemical balance, and smoothing out differences. They are the hardest oils to detect in the finished blend, as they tend to do their job and "integrate," becoming invisible. One can sense their work, but can't remember their personality as easily as those of the other oils.

Top notes: These are the flamboyant, bombastic, young and restless bunch. They make a quick and strong presence and disappear so that you can't catch them. They are important because they add that unforgettable spark to the blend that makes it interesting. Be careful with them, as they are sharp, penetrating, and very volatile. They will likely be the ones to give you the most trouble.

The classification of oils for blending does not always coincide. Following is my own classification of the oils included in this book:

Base notes: Frankincense, jasmine, rose, sandalwood, and ylang ylang.

Middle notes: Geranium, neroli, lemon, clary sage, rosemary, and tea tree.

Top notes: Basil, bergamot, chamomile, and lavender.

Personal Perfumes

In the early eighties, beginning my path as an aromatherapy practitioner, I became aware of the potential that perfumes have in therapy, especially if the perfume making is done with true botanical oils, which have therapeutic properties.

I went to live in Brazil for a couple of years and set myself to have sessions and catalog as many personal preferences of aromas from essential oils as I could, with as many people as I could.

I have the firm belief that people can access emotional healing and mental harmony by using a personalized perfume, one that contains all of their best memories with favorable emotional content. So that is how I began to blend perfumes—by making personal perfumes for clients that I considered "patients." I created sessions in which clients go through a screening process where they smell and grade between 24 and 30 essential oils and absolutes.

This method uses a kit containing aromas in a set of vials, into which I placed small pieces of blotter paper containing a drop or two of each essential oil, and a chart to note the preferences. The different smells were screened from -2 for sure rejection, -1 for dislike, 0 for a feeling of neutrality, +1 for positive reaction and +2 for a definite preference. After creating this chart by smelling the aromas, the client turns the scores over to me. At this point, I create the perfume according to their preferences and achieving the right balance between base, middle, and top notes.

I find this to be a unique method, not only because there is nothing more emotional and aromatically empowering to an individual than a custom-made perfume, but also because the process itself is therapeutic to the client and educational for the aromatherapy perfumer. I have learned so much about people's personalities and their problems, what seems to empower them and how all this relates to the character of the different oils, in a perspective of psycho-aromatherapy. When I am blending a personal perfume for someone, I feel that person telling me how to compose a certain harmony having to do with their very best, then I put it in a bottle.

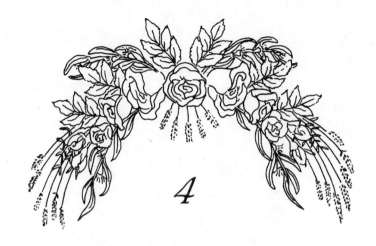

4

Cosmetic Aromatherapy

Exotic Kitchen Recipes

What is holistic about aromatherapy skin care?

Nourishment for the skin.

Healing for the soul.

Relaxation for the mind.

Do it yourself for self-empowerment and creative stimulation.

These three levels—nourishment, healing, and relaxation—are connected. The skin, being the outer and largest organ of the body, is the best representation for the overall health of the body. The health condition of the body, in its turn, is represented by the harmonious balance of all parts of the individual: the body, the emotions and the mind. When one is at risk of being out of balance, so are all the other connecting parts. The use of essential oils on the skin is also the use of essential oils on the emotions and mind. The differences in skin type are also differences in the emotional and mental makeup of each individual. So, fine aromatherapy skin care, by conscious intent, will address all aspects of an individual. Ideally, the person practicing aromatherapy will make personalized skin care treatments.

Cosmetic Aromatherapy

I am an advocate of kitchen cosmetics. They may not be as easy to apply or have as long a shelf life or the fantastic claims that the sophisticated new technology cosmetics do, but the benefits of fresh food for your skin, the personal creative involvement in your skin care, which gives one emotional empowerment and is more economical, by far surpasses the benefit of commodity.

Cosmetic companies rely on the sensational advertisement of the use of some of these ingredients in their formulas. Why not use these ingredients while they are pure and unprocessed, containing the maximum of vital energy, and know exactly what we are putting on our skin?

The knowledge that I am sharing with you in the following pages have come from my common sense, intuition, trial and error, constant reading to evaluate books and articles on nutrition, herbalism, beauty, and aromatherapy. I have also learned from classes with wonderful teachers such as Rosemary Gladstar (the author of *Herbal Healing for Women*) and Dr. Kurt Schnaubelt of the Pacific Institute of Aromatherapy, who gave me a terrific start and a lifelong practice of creating experiments and observing different treatments on my skin as well as others' skin. Before starting my aromatherapy practice, I had already been using herbs and food for beauty, and with the addition of essential oils the pleasure and good results have been multiplying!

In 1986, when I worked in the spas of Calistoga, California, as a massage therapist and facialist, I devised a basic natural skin care system using perishable food materials and essential oils. Ever since that time, this system has been evolving to accommodate my skin's changing needs and the needs of friends and family, ranging from teen to mature skin.

My system consists of preparations to address the following functions of skin care: to clean, to moisturize, to nourish, to stimulate, and to heal.

To clean: Use the scrubs as a soap or cleanser substitute to wash the dead cells off of the skin surface daily. Use clay masks for deep pore cleansing once a week.

To moisturize: You need water and oil; use this combination in a homemade cream or milk. If you are a purist, try the same combination in separate steps. First, use a wrung out steamy hot wash cloth, cover the face for a minute to open pores, then spray floral waters or pat it with lukewarm herbal tea. Follow this step with aromatherapy facial oils, massaging face in gentle upward circular strokes over the water until the oils are absorbed; or you can steam the face, then apply oils. The easiest way is to use facial oils immediately after showering, when skin is saturated with water and pores are open. Oily skin does not need daily creams or facial oils; use herbal steams and honey masks with essential oils instead.

To nourish: Use masks made from fresh food containing vitamins, proteins, and minerals—use fruit, nut butters, seaweed, yeast, algae, honey, and herbs. Apply nourishing masks only after skin cleansing.

To stimulate: Use temperature changes to contract and expand blood vessels causing an increase in blood circulation. Alternate hot and cold with a wash cloth or steam the face, then apply herbal cold splash or rosemary water spray. Follow with acupressure points. (See figure 1, page 114.)

For facials, contract blood vessels using clay or astringent herbs, egg whites, and essential oils; expand with steam and calming facial oils.

Use this to stimulate skin when it is sluggish, dull, or discolored.

To heal: Use essential oil blends with carrier oils or nut milks, herbs, honey, and vitamin E.

Heal skin when skin has acne, is irritated, inflamed, tired or is blemished.

The basic skin care regimen is to clean and moisturize once or twice a day; do deep pore cleansing and nourishing once a week.

The complete facial, done once a month in the following order of application, consists of the following steps.

The scrub, to prepare skin surface for facial.

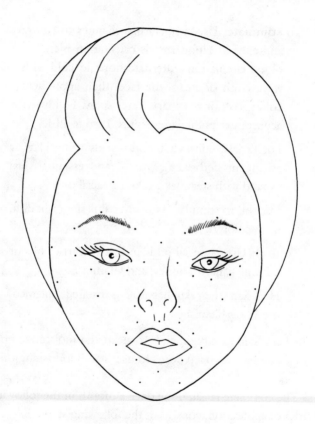

Figure 1. Accupressure points.

A clay mask for deep pore cleansing (use your clay of choice and mix with enough water to make a smooth cream. Add 4 to 6 drops of essential oils according to skin type and mix with water, making a smooth cream). Let the mask dry completely before the herbal steam.

To do an herbal steam, place a handful of herbs in bowl and cover the herbs with half a bowl of boiling water. Cover the bowl with a bath towel for a few seconds; close your eyes, and slide your face into steam just above bowl with towel sealed around your head. Stay under the towel until the steam cools. You can blow on the water to speed the rising of steam. You can also use essential oils in the water. In this case, use only a drop or less of oils and stir the water.

After steaming, wipe off clay with a steamy, hot, wrung-out wash cloth until clay is completely removed, using gentle, circular, upward strokes (see diagram 2, page 116). Rinse with lukewarm water. Now your pores are deeply clean and ready to absorb the vital fresh food in the nourishing masks (see recipes, page 129).

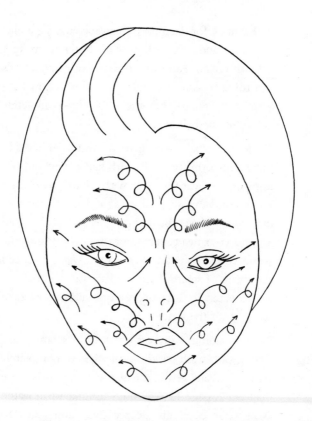

Figure 2. Use upward strokes to cleanse face.

Moisturize skin with combination of facial oils and herbal or floral water spray, facial cream or milk.

The final step in this regimen is to stimulate acupressure points and splash with cold herbal tea or spray with floral waters. Allow skin to air dry.

The following recipes are some of those I have tested and reworked for the last twelve years. The ingredients described on the following pages are to be applied in the recipes, which are a set of simple and more complex formulas for daily use and aromatherapy facials. These recipes illustrate some of the results we can obtain with homemade cosmetics once we begin to experiment with doing it ourselves. Study this information, try mixing some of these formulas, and then create your own!

Before choosing a recipe or ingredient for mixing your own preparation, determine the skin type you're working with. Dry skin feels taut. Normal skin feels smooth and supple. Oily skin feels greasy all over and is sometimes blemished by pimples and acne. Mixed skin is a normal skin with shiny/oily areas such as the nose and chin. Treat mixed skin as separate parts: treat oily areas with applications for oily skin and treat the remaining areas as normal skin. Sensitive skin develops rashes easily and is delicate. Inflamed skin has acne, redness, and abrasion.

Ingredient Descriptions

Following are some of the alive and edible elements of the homemade skin care recipes in this book, all available in good health food stores.

Almonds: Alkaline food rich in calcium, magnesium, protein, and fat. Can be used on the skin as a milk, butter, or pulp mixed with essential oils. Buy organic nuts.

Almond Milk recipe: To produce one cup of almond milk, soak twenty medium to large-size almonds in drinking water over night, or pour boiling water over almonds and let it sit for 30 minutes. (This method makes it easier to peel almonds prior to blending, if so desired.) Next, drain the water and put almonds in a cup of fresh water and set on high speed in a blender for 2 minutes or until it reaches a smooth creamy consistency. Squeeze pulp through a fine sieve or through a cotton cloth bag (the gold coffee strainers work great). Now you have the precious milk. If you don't use the milk immediately, refrigerate it, as it is energy-packed and highly perishable. It will last about three days if refrigerated. The remaining solid mass is the pulp, which can be used in scrubs for face and body. For sensitive skin, I recommend peeling the almonds before blending. This may be quite a bit of work, but I guarantee the results! All skin types.

Aloe Vera: This is a mucilageneous plant. Use gel or juice for cooling, soothing and healing to skin abrasion, rashes, burns. If you have a plant, open the succulent leaf and use the gel inside, or you can buy aloe vera juice bottled with at least 95 percent pure juice.

Black Currant Seed Oil: Contains fatty acids high in gamma-linoleic acid, a substance that supports the reconstruction of damaged skin and other cell membranes. Good to add to healing formulas for acne and inflamed skin. Use combined with vitamin E, in small quantities. Keep refrigerated to avoid rancidity.

Borage Oil: Has the same properties as black currant seed oil. Keep refrigerated.

Brewer's Yeast: Microscopic plant called *Saccharomyces Cerevisiae*. It is a food powder or flakes containing the entire B vitamin complex and concentrated protein with all amino acids. Nutrient. All skin types.

Clay: Deep cleanser of the pores. All clays have negative ionic charge and pull harmful positive ions from the toxins being eliminated by the skin. Absorbs debris and oil, which is washed off the skin with the clay after it dries. Clays, when mixed in water, have drawing action as they dry—from the high swelling and shrinking factor—making skin contract. Clays occur under or on the ground all around the world and can have different colors according to their mineral content: red, black and brown clays are iron rich; the green clays are copper rich; the blue clays, which are cooling and good to use in inflamed skin conditions, are cobalt rich; still other clays are pure white. All clays have drawing and drying action, some more than others. After clay therapy, always moisturize the skin as it is drying.

Bentonite is the most drawing clay, recommended for oily skin, as it easily absorbs excess oil on the skin. Unfortunately it is the most difficult clay to mix and to wash off.

Kaolin is my favorite clay. It is an easy to mix, all-purpose hydrous aluminum silicate. It is a creamy, fine white clay used in making porcelain and is perfect for normal, dry, and sensitive skin for its smooth, clean, and gentle drawing feel. It's very versatile and it lends itself well to mixing with any texture ingredient, such as sticky honey or fibrous fruit pulp.

Comfrey: A very healing, mucilaginous herb. The root has a high content of alantoin, a substance that supports the building of new cells. Dry or fresh leaves can be used in facial steams and powdered leaves can be used as healing poultices mixed with honey. Skin type: inflamed/acne.

Enzymes: Needed for all processes of metabolism. Anti-oxidant agents and catalysts, aids other cells in eliminating, coagulating, building, fixing cells, and decomposing. Enzymes attack waste material and can help protect the skin against harmful bacteria. Use rejuvilac, an enzyme-rich liquid for mixing into facial masks or as a digestive drink.

Rejuvilac recipe: Soak organic grains—such as wheat or dried fruits—in at least twice the volume of spring water at warm temperature, until tiny bubbles form and float to surface (approximately 24 hours). Drain and refrigerate. It will keep for many weeks and will smell foul when too old.

Evening Primrose Oil: Skin cell restoration aid. Holds the highest percentage of gamma-linoleic acid, which supports the reconstruction of damaged cell membranes. It has a therapeutic action in many of the body systems, such as circulatory, digestive, and the neuro-endocrine complex. Keep refrigerated. All skin types.

Honey: Natural bactericide, helps equalize pH acid/alkaline balance on the skin. Can be used as a cleanser, especially on oily skin when no oil or milks are desired. Honey is also an emollient, softening agent, full of life force and energizing to the skin as it creates the perfect base for powdered herbs and food stuffs in scrubs. Use unprocessed honey. Soap substitute. All skin types.

Hydrolates/Hydrosols or floral water sprays: Hydrolates are the resulting water from the condensation of steam distillation after the essential oil has been removed. Hydrolates are saturated with hydrophilic compounds that are present in plants, but not in the essential oils. These compounds are water soluble. The carboxylic acids present here are not found in essential oils and are the most calming therapeutic elements found in the plants. Harsh components—such as aggressive terpine hydrocarbons alcohols found in essential oils—are dissolved in the hydrosols due to their hydroxyl group. Beneficial properties of terpines and sesquiterpines alcohols include antiseptic, lymphatic decongestant, tonic stimulant uses.

Hydrolates are totally safe for all skin and eye care applications, including inflamed and infected conditions. Chamomile is the mildest, rose the most astringent, and neroli the most hydrating. Lavender can be considered all-purpose.

Nut Butters: These are nutrients that can also work as emollients for the skin, containing protein, fat, and important minerals for the skin such as calcium, a nerve tranquilizer; magnesium, which helps absorption of calcium and activates some enzymes; and iron. Choose from almond, Brazil nut, cashews, macadamia, and vitamin E-rich sesame seed butter—tahini. Always mix these butters with honey. All skin types.

Rose Hip Seed Oil: Also known as *Rose rubiginosa* or *Rosa mosqueta,* an important oil from the seed of a South American variety of the wild rose. Similar to evening primrose oil in properties, it is very rich in gammalinoleic acid and prevents skin cell membrane damage. All skin types, particularly useful for skin affected by premature aging.

Seaweed: Edible sea vegetable with a high concentration of minerals that are important in skin care. Nutrient rich in iodine, which stimulates circulation; calcium for reducing nerve ending irritability; and iron for toning facial muscles. Kelp powder and dulse flakes are best suited for skin use. All skin types.

Slippery Elm: An herbal powder with mucilaginous properties. Softens and helps soothe inflammation and infections of the mucous membranes. A protector agent. It is good mixed with fibrous materials such as powdered dry herbs in scrubs. Skin types: dry and sensitive; inflamed/acne.

Spirulina: Anti-oxidant. A green algae in powder form. It is a concentrated food containing chlorophyll, a blood purifier. Contains 60 percent protein; vitamin A, which protects the skin from infections and all the B vitamins, which are the vitamins with the most important organic functions for the skin. Very powerful nutrient for facial masks. All skin types.

Vitamin E: Anti-oxidant. Helps eradicate free radicals, those unbalanced molecules containing unpaired electrons that seek electrons in cell membranes and body-building proteins causing alteration in molecular structure creating an unbalanced chain reaction. Vitamin E can be used in homemade cosmetics as a natural preservative. All skin types.

Essential Oils and Skin Types

Normal skin: Chamomile, blue and Roman; clary sage; geranium; lavender; neroli; rose; sandalwood.

Oily skin: Clary sage, eucalyptus, lavender, lemon, peppermint, rose, rosemary, tea tree.

Dry/sensitive skin: Chamomile, blue and Roman; frankincense; lavender; neroli.

Inflamed/acne: Chamomile, blue and Roman; clary sage; lavender; lemon; neroli; rose; tea tree.

Mature skin: Clary sage, frankincense, jasmine, lavender, neroli, rose, sandalwood.

Herbs and Skin Types

Use these in steams and scrubs with the appropriate skin types.

Normal skin: Chamomile, lavender, peppermint, rose.

Oily skin: Lavender, peppermint, rose, rosemary, clary sage.

Dry/sensitive skin: Basil, chamomile, comfrey, lavender, mullen.

Acne/Inflamed skin: Chamomile, comfrey, lavender, mullen, rose.

Fruit and Skin Care

Many fruits have special value for nourishing skin applications.

Cucumber: Botanically a fruit, cucumber is an astringent with a toning quality. Contains protein and digestive enzymes. Rich in vitamins A and C and calcium.

Honeydew melon: Skin cleanser rich in vitamins A and C. Can be a substitute for papaya and strawberries in some formulas. Dry skin.

Papaya: Helps activate blood circulation in the capillaries. Contains the enzyme papain, which breaks down protein for better absorption. Contains vitamin A and C. It is a luxurious emollient, softening the skin as it nourishes.

Pineapple: Enzyme-rich juice containing vitamins A and C. Helps sluggish skin activate blood circulation in the capillaries.

Strawberries: Skin cleanser rich in vitamins A and C. Helps skin to eliminate toxins. Pulp has been traditionally used as poultices to alleviate sore eyes.

Tomato: Natural antiseptic. Purifying agent rich in vitamins A and C, calcium, and magnesium. Good for skin blemishes, pimples, and acne.

Exotic Kitchen Recipes

Instructions for preparing some of the ingredients listed in these recipes appear at the beginning of this chapter, beginning on page 118.

Note: *Tanacetum Annuum* is a wonderful oil containing azulene components that I like to use as an alternative to blue chamomile in these formulas. The scent is much more desirable than the common German—or blue—chamomile, *Matricaria recutica*.

The rosemary that I use, which is more appropriate for skin care, is chemotype *Rosemary verbanon*. See the recommendations for essential oil sources on page 238 if you can't find them at a retail store near you.

Scrubs

The scrubs are soap and cleanser substitutes for daily use prior to moisturizing the skin. Apply on wet skin, but avoid getting water into the scrub jar. These scrubs are fairly stable from spoilage, but are best kept away from heat and direct sunlight. These recipes make approximately 1 ounce.

Simple Scrub for All Skin Types

6 drops lavender

2 tablespoons raw honey

2 tablespoons brewer's yeast

Mix lavender into honey, then stir in yeast until the mixture is smooth.

Fancy Scrub for Normal Skin

2 tablespoons dry rose petals

6 macadamia nuts

Essential oils:

    3 drops Roman chamomile

    2 drops lavender

    2 drops clary sage

    1 drop neroli

1 tablespoon dry lavender flowers

1 chamomile tea bag (the Traditionals brand is best)

Honey

You will need a mortar and pestle and a clean coffee or nut grinder or similar implement.

Grind your rose petals to smaller flakes. Grind nuts into fine meal in mortar. Add essential oils to nut meal and mix.

Add nut meal and lavender flowers to the grinder and run it a few times with the ground rose petals until the mixture resembles an even, fine meal; be careful not to overdo it. Pour out the contents from the grinder and mix the chamomile petals from the tea bag into the rest of mix with a small spoon. Save this mix and prepare ½ ounce at a time with equal parts of honey for your daily use. For example, use ¼ ounce mix and ¼ ounce honey. Apply the scrub on wet face with gentle, circular, upwards strokes and rinse with lukewarm water. (See diagram on page 116.)

Simple Scrub for Oily Skin

Essential oils:

- 1 drop peppermint
- 3 drops lavender
- 6 drops lemon

1 tablespoon raw honey

1 teaspoon sesame butter (tahini)

1 teaspoon brewer's yeast

1 teaspoon kelp granules or powder

Pour essential oils into the honey and mix well. Add the tahini. Mix in the dry ingredients last, one at a time, mixing vigorously until smooth. It should have a stiff consistency. Spread it on wet face in circular, upward strokes. Wash off with lukewarm water and a final cold splash.

Simple Scrub for Normal to Oily Skin with Acne and Pimples

  2 chamomile tea bags
  2 tablespoons honey
     Essential oils
        1 drop blue chamomile
        2 drops Roman chamomile
        1 drop lavender

Mix essential oils into a 1-ounce glass jar. Pour honey into the jar, mixing with the oils. Pour contents of tea bags into honey and essential oils and mix until smooth. Apply to the face with gentle, circular, upward strokes on wet face and rinse with lukewarm water.

Fancy Scrub for Inflamed Skin and Acne

  1 tablespoon fresh almond meal (resulting from preparation of almond milk, see recipe, page 118)
  1 tablespoon comfrey powder

    1 teaspoon mullen powder
       Essential oils:
          6 drops lemon
          4 drops tea tree
          2 drops rosemary verbanon
    1 tablespoon aloe vera juice
    1 tablespoon honey

Powder herbs in grinder, then push through a sieve or strainer. Mix essential oils into honey. Mix all wet ingredients, then mix powders into wet ingredients. Apply it on dry skin with gentle, circular, upward stokes. Rinse with lukewarm water. It will keep three days if refrigerated.

Facial Oils

The following formulas will make 15 milliliters of facial oil. (15 milliliters = 1 tablespoon = 300 drops).

For each recipe, mix essential oils first in a small glass bottle, then pour in the other oils and shake. The mixture will not go rancid if you keep it in a cool shaded place. Use after a scrub, showering, steam, or herbal/floral spray. See appendix for recommended sources for obtaining your materials.

Normal Skin

5 milliliters hazelnut or grapeseed oil
8 milliliters rice bran oil
2 capsules evening primrose oil
2 capsules vitamin E
2 drops frankincense
2 drops rose otto
1 drop neroli
1 drop Roman chamomile

Dry/Sensitive Skin

8 milliliters aloe vera oil
5 milliliters avocado oil
1 capsule vitamin E
1 milliliter rose hip oil
4 drops sandalwood
2 drops Roman chamomile
1 drop lavender
1 drop blue chamomile

Milks

See the recipe for fresh almond milk, which is used in both recipes, on page 118. Refrigerate milks to make them last a few days.

Soothing Moisture for
Inflamed Skin and Rashes

1 ounce almond milk
2 drops lavender
1 drop blue chamomile

Mix essential oils into a clean glass container, then pour in almond milk and stir. Blue chamomile will not mix completely in milk, so you must agitate vigorously before applying on skin. Smooth over clean or steamed skin with circular, upward strokes. Allow to dry and do not rinse face.

Healing Milk for Oily Skin with Acne

1 ounce almond milk
4 drops lemon oil
2 drops clary sage
1 drop lavender
1 drop rose otto

Mix these essential oils into a clean glass container, then stir in milk, following with vigorous shaking. Smooth over steamed skin with circular, upward, gentle stokes. Let dry and do not rinse.

Frequently, oily skin and skin with acne are brutally treated with harsh chemicals and intense scrubbing. Acne often happens in very emotionally sensitive people, to whom the practice of self-acceptance and love is an issue. Rose otto is a luxury that contributes to soothing the emotions and, at the same time, is a mild astringent helping to correct excessive oil on the skin.

Masks

These are the most vital, perishable, and luxurious skin applications. Use organically grown ingredients if possible and avoid mixing into containers made of aluminum or wood. Wait for your pamper day to mix these, when you can take time out and treat your skin to super nourishment while you relax. These nourishing masks are at their best on the day they are mixed; however, they will still be effective for one or two more days if refrigerated. Use a mask by itself, or as part of a facial. You can use the leftover mixture on your body after exfoliating with a fiber brush.

Emerald Moss

This is an anti-inflammatory aromatic live green gel meant
to nourish inflamed/acne skin. Oily and normal skin may
use this formula as a firming gel.

  1 tablespoon comfrey root
  ¼ cup boiling water
10 almonds
  1 tablespoon ripe tomato pulp
  1 teaspoon spirulina
  1 teaspoon slippery elm powder
     Essential oils:
       3 drops lemon oil
       2 drops tea tree
       2 drops rosemary verbanon
       1 drop blue chamomile
       1 drop peppermint

Soak comfrey root in the ¼ cup of boiling water while
you prepare the almond milk by the following quick
method: Pour more boiling water on almonds and let sit
until water is lukewarm. Drain water out and push almonds
out of skins. Place all 10 peeled almonds in the blender to
wait while you prepare all other ingredients.

Strain tomato pulp into a bowl, separating seeds and skin aside. Measure 1 tablespoon of tomato pulp and place it in a bowl. Mix spirulina into the tomato pulp with a small spoon until smooth, then add the slippery elm, mixing continuously until smooth. Add essential oils and keep stirring. Stir comfrey root water, then drain through a strainer, adding this mucilaginous water to the almonds in the blender. Blend at high speed until homogenous.

Strain the mixture to collect ¼ cup of liquid; you can add a little water through the pulp to complete this measurement if needed.

Add this almond/comfrey liquid very slowly, continuously stirring, to the rest of recipe until homogeneous. You should end up with a smooth, translucent, green gel; let it sit for a minute before applying on dry skin. Let mask dry completely before removing with a steaming hot, wrung out wash cloth, using gentle, upward, circular strokes. Rinse face in cool water and air dry. This is also a good formula for acne on the back or other body parts.

Papaya and Almond Sea Foam

Luxurious nourishing mask for dry and sensitive skins.

- 1 teaspoon dulse flakes
- 10 presoaked almonds
- ½ cup of rejuvilac (page 122)
- 1 tablespoon papaya pulp
- ½ teaspoon slippery elm
- ½ teaspoon honey
- 1 capsule vitamin E
  Essential oils:
  - 6 drops sandalwood
  - 2 drops neroli
  - 1 drop Roman chamomile
  - 1 drop blue chamomile

Rinse dulse flakes in warm water and place with the almonds into the rejuvilac. Blend for two minutes at high speed, strain, and let it sit while you prepare the other ingredients.

Mix papaya pulp, slippery elm, honey, and vitamin E. Mix essential oils into the rejuvilac mixture, then pour it into the rest of mixture, stirring until smooth. Apply mask to dry skin and let it dry completely before wiping off with a steaming hot wrung-out wash cloth with gentle, circular, upward strokes. Rinse with lukewarm water, ending with a final cool splash or floral spray.

Strawberry Rose Glow

Nourishing and calming mask for normal skin.

- 1 tablespoon strawberry pulp
- 1 tablespoon barley flower
- ½ teaspoon fresh almond milk (page 118)
- ½ teaspoon rejuvilac (page 122)
- ½ teaspoon honey
  Essential oils:
    - 2 drops rose otto
    - 1 drop lavender
    - 1 drop neroli

Mix strawberry pulp with the barley flour. Mix almond milk with the rejuvilac. Mix honey with essential oils.

Blend all three mixtures and stir until smooth. Apply on dry face and let it dry completely. Wipe off with a steaming hot wrung-out wash cloth with gentle, circular, upward strokes. Rinse with lukewarm water, then with a final cool splash or spray.

Hot Oil Hair Treatment

This treatment opens the hair follicles, giving the essential oils a chance to work deep down to the roots, stimulating circulation. It leaves hair pliable and shiny. Use once a month to maintain healthy hair and diminish the proliferation of split ends.

Normal, Dry and Damaged Hair

1 tablespoon jojoba oil
½ tablespoon avocado oil
½ tablespoon aloe vera oil
Essential oils:
   10 drops rosemary
    6 drops lavender
    3 drops geranium
    1 drop peppermint

Mix vegetable oils in a double boiler or a fondue crock pot and heat to about 70 degrees F. Remove from heat and add essential oils, stirring to mix. For long hair, dip ends of brushed hair into the hot oil and carefully spread oil to rest of hair, massaging upward towards scalp. Put hair into a plastic cap and cover with a warm towel. Leave for at least

30 minutes, brushing again with a comb and shampooing twice to remove all oil. For short hair, apply oil to hair as hot as your hands will take and follow the same procedure as described above. Makes one application.

Baby Care
Infant Massage Oil

¼ ounce aloe vera oil
½ ounce rice bran oil
¼ ounce hazelnut oil
Essential oils:
    3 drops blue chamomile
    7 drops lavender

Makes one ounce. The full ounce can be made with rice bran oil or another carrier oil alone.

For more further information on homemade cosmetics, see appendix.

5

Medical Aromatherapy

A Travel Kit

Therapies using essential oils are not to be understood with the same attitude of "instant results" in the way it is expected of allopathic medicine. However, in my own life, I have noticed amazingly fast results at certain times.

In medical aromatherapy, essential oils are ingested, used as suppositories, inhaled, or applied on the skin—on the whole body, or localized areas—through massage. The aromatic molecules penetrate the body, entering the blood stream through the skin by massage, into the lungs by inhalation and into the digestive system by ingestion or suppository application.

Certain oils can cross the blood-brain barrier and reach the brain tissue, causing damage to nerves and tissue. However, these toxic oils can be used therapeutically, which is the reason education in medical aromatherapy is crucial before using aromatherapy as a system for self-treatment.

There are doctors, among whom are Dr. Jean Valnet, Dr. Jean Claude Lapraz, Dr. Daniel Pénoël, and research scientist Pierre Franchomme, who are experts in the medical use of essential oils and tour Europe and the United States teaching medical aromatherapy. In France, aromatherapy is a course offered in pharmaceutical and medical schools.

One of the most important thing that happens when one uses aromatherapy is that it puts the individual in touch with a form of holistic healing that addresses more than the physical body in a very tangible way through smell. For example, lemon oil is a strong antiseptic, serving the purpose of protecting the body's respiratory system from infection. As the lemon oil is addressing the respiratory infection, it simultaneously has an effect on the nervous system, since one of its properties is to act as a sedative to the nervous system. So, by affecting the emotions to calm the individual during the condition, the mind will settle and be directed to another experience through the olfactory system. The aroma of the lemon oil will rest the mind from discomfort and let the body do the healing.

This constitutes a pleasurable way to deal with illness that, in the long run, pays off on many levels. There are currently a few physicians using aromatherapy in their practices.

Some oils can be applied without dilution. Among those, lavender and tea tree are two of the most important oils because of their wide range of properties. Some oils are safe to apply neat, without dilution, to certain tissue but not on other tissue. Even oils that are non-toxic can aggravate and cause discomfort to certain tissue. For example, you can use rosemary inside your nostrils as a decongestant, but it is inappropriate to use it neat on the armpits, as it could cause a burning sensation. One can use lavender on an open cut on the limbs, but not on the vaginal tissue.

Citrus oils, including bergamot, should never be used in preparations involving sun exposure, as they are photo-sensitive and can permanently stain the skin.

Preparations for babies and pregnant women need different considerations, as well.

A good habit to develop to test for sensitivity is to always first apply a blend on a small area of the skin before applying oils, even diluted, on a full body massage or on a larger area of the body.

Hypotensive individuals should avoid the oils that activate blood circulation such as basil, peppermint, or rosemary.

There is so much to know about the medical uses of essential oils that a book such as this one cannot possibly cover all the necessary facts. Please refer to the appendix for books on the subject and education sources.

Medicinal Travel Kit

Following is a small and safe essential oil kit I use for simple therapies while I am traveling. I acquired this medical aromatherapy knowledge from studying with Pierre Franchomme and Dr. Pénoël and experimenting for a number of years.

Essential oils in the kit, 5 milliliters each: basil, bergamot, blue chamomile, clary sage, eucalyptus, frankincense, geranium, lavender, lemon, neroli, peppermint, roman chamomile, rose otto, rosemary, sandalwood, tea tree, ylang ylang.

Abdominal pain and intestinal gas: Use 6 drops of peppermint, variety *Mentha piperita* only, in ½ ounce of vegetable oil. Massage the area every two hours and drink peppermint tea. Four drops of *Mentha piperita* can be ingested or used as suppository, inside gelatin capsules, up to 2 times each day.

Aching muscles: Massage oil of 15 drops of lavender and two drops of blue chamomile in 1 ounce of vegetable oil.

Athlete's foot: Dab tea tree neat, onto the foot, every hour.

Burns, cuts, insect bites: Dab lavender, neat, on the affected area.

Bladder irritations: These therapies will provide relief and comfort to a bladder infection and keep the infection from getting worse. If an allopathic drug is used, such as antibiotics, these essential oil therapies can be used at the same time. It is very good and strengthening to keep these oils flowing through the bladder and stay connected with your plant oil allies.

Drink 2 to 3 quarts per day of bergamot-tea tree tea (page 156). Multiply the recipe to make a gallon for a sitz bath before bedtime. To cure a bladder infection, one must use thyme, oregano, and savory, with correct chemotypes and prescription. (See *L'aromatherapie exactament* by Pénoël and Franchome.)

Boils and skin infection: Support tissue with application of lavender or tea tree. Both can be applied, undiluted, directly on inflamed tissue. This will keep the area clean, and keep infection from spreading further, supporting the formation of scar tissue. If skin is very inflamed and fairly red, add one drop of blue chamomile to the lavender or tea tree. If you insist, it won't persist.

Congested sinuses and respiratory infections: For inhalation, apply 1 drop eucalyptus, 2 drops rosemary, and 5 drops lemon to steamy hot water and inhale as much as possible under a towel with closed eyes. Repeat this treatment every 4 hours. It is also nice to mix two parts lemon with one part eucalyptus and use a couple of drops on a cloth to inhale during the course of the day. Drink tea tree-lemon tea (page 157).

Diarrhea: Drink chamomile-basil tea (page 157). Three drops of lemon and 3 drops of *Mentha piperita* can be taken in gelatin capsules twice a day or applied as suppository.

Food poisoning: Mix 4 drops of lemon into a teaspoon of honey and pour hot water over it to make tea. Drink up to three cups a day. This tea can also be used as a preventive to protect one from contracting contagious infections from others, such as in seasonal flu epidemics.

Herpes simplex: Mix one part eucalyptus with one part tea tree and apply with fingertip neat on the sore every hour. Use vitamin E between applications to support tissue while it is being dried up by the constant application of the oils. It cuts the edge of pain and heals in one week instead of two. If you have rose otto and geranium, this is an even more efficient therapy for herpes simplex. Follow the same instructions given above, just substitute the oils. This second combination is much milder on the lip tissue. It may even have a faster healing time, and the vitamin E can be nice, but it is not as necessary.

Headaches: Apply lavender with a drop of peppermint on temples, on the back of the neck, and between nose and upper lip. At night, put two drops of lavender on your pillow. Drink lavender tea (page 157) or precious flower tea (page 158).

Insomnia: Apply a couple drops of lavender on your pillow.

Mental fatigue: Do a hot foot bath with 6 drops of rosemary. Rub a couple of undiluted drops of peppermint between the palms of your hands, cup your hands over nose, and inhale deeply. Avoid getting the peppermint in your eyes. Peppermint cannot hurt you, but it will deliver a burning sensation to your eyes for quite some time.

Nausea and motion sickness: Use lavender, basil, or peppermint for inhalation by pouring a couple of drops in a handkerchief to sniff during bouts of motion sickness or other types of nausea.

PMS and uterine cramps: Mix 1 drop of blue chamomile and 2 drops of lavender with 5 drops of clary sage into ½ ounce of vegetable oil. Massage the mixture on lower abdomen. Avoid this treatment during pregnancy. Drink precious flower tea (page 158).

Sunburn: Mix 10 drops of lavender into ½ ounce of aloe vera oil or almond oil and apply gently on skin.

Vaginal dryness: Mix 2 parts jojoba oil and 1 part melted cocoa butter to make 1 ounce. Add to this mixture 3 drops sandalwood and 1 drop geranium. Stir while warm to an even mix. Allow to cool to solidify. Smooth the mixture with fingers over tissue, two times a day and before intercourse. Completely safe. You can use one drop of neroli instead of one drop of geranium.

Making Essential Oil Teas

I have developed a habit of making tea using essential oils. Although it may be an acquired taste for some, and involves a previous dilution into a tablespoon of vodka, brandy, wine, or other alcohol prior to inverting essential oils into water, tea is a great way to use essential oils for simple therapies while traveling.

Essential oils in my suggested travel kit that are good for tea preparation are basil, bergamot, roman chamomile, lavender, lemon, neroli, rose, and tea tree. While traveling, I find it advantageous to use oils instead of herbs, because essential oils do not have a shelf life like herbs do, and they occupy a lot less space. I have always found it valuable to have a few 5-milliliter bottles of oil in my carry-on while flying. I ask the flight attendant for some hot water to prepare my tea in flight. (Avoid using styrofoam cups; essential oils will carve holes in the cup. Choose glass or porcelain.) This practice has always made my flight more pleasant and energized.

The environment of an aircraft, combined with the fact that our bodies are so far from the earth, is depleting to our systems. I have found it to be a great help to have the life-giving qualities of plant oils close at hand, as allies, during my travels. Often, people sitting next to me also enjoy the aroma, and I frequently end up answering questions and giving a mini-lecture on essential oils to the curious neighbors.

Essential oils in the correct measure can be mixed into sugar and alcohol and dispersed in the hot water enough for one to have a pleasant drink. However, the essential oils will not completely dissipate into the water, so expect to see oil floating on the surface of your tea—some more than others, depending on the degree of volatility of each oil—but if the recipe is done carefully, this should not be a problem. The more volatile oils, such as lavender, peppermint, or rose, have a fine dispersion. The citrus oils lemon and bergamot require stirring teach prior to drinking it each time. Good teas to drink while flying are basil, roman chamomile, lavender, lemon, neroli, peppermint, rose otto, and tea tree. My favorite tea for supporting my digestive system during flight is a combination of roman chamomile with basil, or just plain basil. To sleep, lavender with roman chamomile or rose otto are effective teas.

Preparing Essential Oil Teas

Mix the recipe of the desired oil into one or two teaspoons of sugar, mixing vigorously to distribute essential oil into the sugar evenly. Slowly add one tablespoon of vodka and then one cup of hot water, pouring hot water over sugar slowly, mixing continuously. Oils will not disperse completely in the water, but the dispersion after careful mixing is pleasant enough to drink. Citrus oils may require stirring prior to drinking. One can use honey or maple syrup instead of sugar, but it will be a little more difficult to do the mixing.

Essential Oil Tea Recipes

These recipes have been tested, using oils completely safe for digestion.

Mix the appropriate oils with 1 or 2 tablespoons of sugar; 1 tablespoon of vodka, brandy, or wine; and 8 ounces of hot water (one cup) as described above.

Bladder Irritation

3 drops bergamot oil
6 drops tea tree oil

Colds, Flu, and Respiratory Infections

2 drops lemon oil

6 drops tea tree oil

Diarrhea

2 drops basil oil

1 drop Roman chamomile oil

Flatulence

1 drop peppermint oil

Insomnia

1 drop lavender oil

½ drop Roman chamomile oil

or use a simple lavender tea:

2 drops lavender oil

Nausea and Motion Sickness

1 drop peppermint oil

2 drops basil oil

PMS, Anxiety, Nervous Tension

Use either precious flower tea or rose otto tea.

Precious Flower Tea

    2 drops lavender oil
    1 drop rose otto
    1 drop neroli oil *(optional)*
    2 tablespoons sugar
    1 tablespoon vodka, brandy, or wine
    4 cups hot water

Rose Otto Tea

    1 drop rose otto
    2 cups water
    2 teaspoons sugar
    1 tablespoon vodka, brandy, or wine

These two teas are sedatives and they work great hot or chilled. Essential oil teas, especially the precious flower tea, mature nicely in the refrigerator overnight.

Try the tea chilled, on a hot afternoon with ice, and a sprig of peppermint. Voila! A fantastic wine substitute. Therapeutic properties will remain, and it is a very exotic party drink.

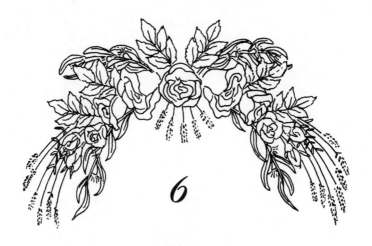

6

Psycho-Aromatherapy

Case Studies

*T*his is my chapter. The one I had to learn alone in order to write it. It is also the one in which my heart is at its fullest, and it is my present contribution to psycho-aromatherapy and vibrational medicine. The two are marvelously connected, something that I will explain in chapter 8.

My interest in psycho-aromatherapy began through my work with personalized perfumes for clients who would tell me how empowering and therapeutic the scents of their personal perfumes were to them. I began to realize the healing possibilities that scent can play in therapies involving the use of memory and focus to address mental blocks caused by a past bad experience.

The relationship between smell and memory holds a tremendous potential for a healer or therapist working with the emotional and mental states of an individual. The limbic system, the area of the brain processing memory and emotion, is also where the cells that process the information coming from the nerve endings connecting to the olfactory bulb are located. Memory and emotion are not associated to odor processing by chance. We need information from our sense of smell to access behavior we may need to apply. One simple example is detecting a decomposing smell on a portion of food prior to eating it. From that acknowledgment comes the decision to discard the food, knowing that it can upset the digestive system. If our sense of smell was not functioning properly, we would miss that important information and eat food that would make us sick. The next time the same type of food is served, our "smell brain" will unconsciously process the memory of the previous smell and automatically do a smell comparison with the previous smell memory and signal OK if the decomposing smell is not present this time. This is one example of the myriad subtle ways that we are ordinarily functioning with odor and memory processing, which most times happens unconsciously.

If one wishes to use this function consciously, as an aid in therapies, there are numerous ways in which this can be done. One way is to use a positive association in order to achieve a certain result. In hospitals, a technique is used for giving a child in the operating room the smell of chocolate at the time of anesthesia. This distracts the fear by creating a feeling with a positive association.

The relationship between memory and odor consciously used in therapies has at least a couple of levels of association.

The healer or therapist who is bringing an individual a smell with the intention of creating a good change holds the first level of this association. The healer automatically represents a positive, caring, and powerful influence. This first level of association opens the door.

When the scent merges with memory, one can respond to the second level of association, which is with the smell itself. A given image can be programmed with a specific intention and a smell.

This second level provides an environment for the focus that will create the emotional change that is sought.

Intention, although a non-physical element, plays an important role for those working with energy and its subtle modalities for effecting change.

Here we must again speak holistically of the ways in which the different parts of our being are connected and cannot be separated. The healer or therapist using this type of therapy must enjoy being a little like a detective and must penetrate further than the body to find out what is going on with the mind and emotions of the person being treated. Discovering what the empowering smells coming from this person's environment are can be important—likes and dislikes contain many clues about what one should or should not use.

The more focused on helping another person, the more the healer's intuition is activated. Knowledge from facts, together with intuitive feelings, creates equations with balanced results.

The choice of which essential oil to use must come from knowledge of how this oil affects the mind, emotions, and body—which can also vary with each individual depending on his or her previous associations, likes, and dislikes.

The goal is to create and help the person register a specific emotional program with an odor association. This can be done consciously, in cases of removing a certain negative mental block that can be creating a illness. Sometimes the smell can be applied alone with no logical mind intervention, as in the case of Marty Winn, detailed below.

The following real life stories serve to illustrate a few of the many ways that therapies using aroma can be helpful.

Marty Winn

General Contractor in his late thirties
Sebastopol, California

Kendra: Marty had a pre-existing heart condition from a car accident a few years earlier. I visited him in the hospital at the time of a second accident, when a school bus collided with his sports car, fracturing eight of his ribs, breaking his femur in six pieces, crushing his kneecap and ankle, and splitting his tibia lengthwise. He had two severe skull fractures and his collarbone and sternoclavicular and rotator cuff joints were broken. Marty was in traction and on morphine when I came to visit him at the beginning of his second week in the hospital. This man was in serious trouble—a big strong guy who could normally lift 300 pounds over his head with no trouble at all was now in a hospital bed unable to lift his own arm, waiting for the life and death decision of his second surgery.

The hospital personnel were so intensely busy trying to fix his body that my feeling when I arrived was that they had forgotten Marty all together. From my perspective, I knew immediately that he needed desperate help getting his mind to focus, and healing his emotions was as important as healing his body.

In his situation, Marty did not need any kind of explanation about the therapy I was about to do with him because his mind was saturated with life and death issues and his body was in such bad shape that an explanation seemed absolutely inappropriate. The wordless aromatic experience was all I perceived necessary to address his emotional situation. I used a strongly sedative blend made from rose otto, neroli, and lavender, which I placed inside a crystal pendant (see page 205) hanging from the metal apparatus reaching just above his nose.

Marty: As I was absolutely helpless, lying there wondering if I was going to live or die, I was looking for emotional contact. I was not getting that in the hospital. I remember the aromatic smell. First I kind of liked it, but after a while I had judgment. This was not some kind of Wild Musk Splash cologne or something!

I knew it was essential oils, and I didn't believe in therapeutic properties or anything. I think my emotional bond with Kendra made me trust something that I normally would have thought to be off the wall and disconnected with what was going on.

The fragrance was extremely different. All of a sudden there was a whole new world I could be in and exit my body. Now I was getting something for me. It was like an escape. Lying there, the TV on, I was in a daze from all the drugs, held together by stitches and pins, connected to hoses and tubes—I needed another space to be in. With this little fragrant crystal, I could close my eyes, take great deep breaths and smell this aroma that was putting me in a euphoric state. It made me feel like I could leave my body and heighten my ability to be able to check my mind out from the pain and check into a state where I was emotionally aware without being emotional. I felt myself inside saying: *I am all right, I am going to be OK*. It gave me a positive dimension, it strengthened my emotions enough to face surgery, and as a result, my recovery was a lot faster than expected. I had that crystal with me until after I went home. It supported me emotionally much more then anything or anybody. I could lie there, cover my face, breathe deeply and go into another world. It was better than drugs or even prayers. I would come back energized and ready to repair my body. I was rather surprised in what I received in this little piece of jewelry.

Carla Dykes
Young mother in her twenties
Sebastopol, California

Kendra: Carla had a physical condition arising from the result of open heart surgery when she was five years old. The surgery had severed nerves and she had no sensation in her left breast. She was pregnant with her second baby, due to be born any minute, and still had her first baby, less then two years old, nursing regularly. She'd had some difficulty nursing her first child, which was especially emotional because she could not feel the let-down reflex in one of the breasts and worried that her baby was not getting enough milk. This created a fear-based block that was building with the second child coming, since there was a good chance she would be nursing two babies at once for a while.

When I saw Carla, we had a session during which we discussed therapy using aromas to help her remove the mental and emotional block. Together, we created visual imagery to represent an opening in the energy of the block, relaxing mind and body. She would focus on the imagery while smelling the aroma of rose otto that I would apply on her breast through massage. We did this a few times, and I left the aromatic crystal with the same smell with her so that she could meditate with it and continue the influence between sessions.

Carla: This therapy using aroma was beneficial to me in terms of comforting me in a stressful time, helping to relax the fear. This initiated a process in me so that a change was possible. It gave me an open perspective to see how I can grow in my ability to trust alternative therapies for my healing. I felt the crystal broaden the spectrum of the healing. The stone and the plant oil combination connected me to a greater natural support system in a time when I needed that. I used the aroma to meditate, and that was very healing.

Dr. David Kent

An M.D. anesthesiologist in his fifties
Santa Rosa, California

Kendra: Dr. Kent had a serious pelvic fracture from an in-line skating accident. Being familiar with the hospital environment, he was comfortable and knew the people attending him. His surgery was successful and he and his surgeon were pretty happy with the results. When I came to visit him, he was in the rehabilitation unit and had developed a condition with a blood clot in his right leg, which had a risk of migrating to his lungs, causing cardiac function and respiratory problems. He is a strong, active man and was hoping for his maximum recovery. It was obvious that his main emotional issue was accepting his "soaking" period in bed, without being able to do much and not knowing how long he would be there. There was apprehension and nervousness regarding the outcome. My input with Dr. Kent was purely intuitive. I felt that his condition was yin, arising from a situation when he was fast moving and had a violent halt. The blood clot developed some days after the surgery. To me, this seemed to match the slowing of movement, causing the yin condition now in his blood circulation. I decided to bring him a blood-colored stone—a red tourmaline with purple hues—with Chinese ginger oil in it, which created a strong yang influence for his electromagnetic field with the intention to focus on creating balance. I told him to use the synergy visualizing the yin and yang balance and the dissolving of the clot.

Dr. Kent: Kendra came to visit at a time when I was waiting for the blood to thin to avoid further complications with the blood clot that had developed after the accident. There was not much I could do but just lie there with very little exercise and wait. She loaned me a heart-shaped pendant with ginger oil in it. I did get in trouble shortly after her visit as the blood clot broke loose and I went to the intensive care unit for a couple of days. Gradually I improved and eventually got out of the hospital I had stayed in for a total of four weeks.

I wore the aromatic stone with the ginger oil most of the time while in the hospital. What I felt with that was an energizing, yet gentle, positive psychological feeling. It was not like having perfume under my nose, but it was there and I could notice it and be aware of it and get a waft from it once in a while. It helped me focus on feeling positive by bringing my attention and my awareness to the healing process, as a reminder to put some energy into the healing. It frequently reminded me to focus on this positive aspect. I did feel that it was a positive, energetic thing and not a hypnotizing, passive, or sleep-inducing thing. When I was alone, it kept bringing my attention back to my body healing by using my own energy.

Something else happened—the ginger smell made a memory pop up of a time, years before, when I was traveling in New Guinea with three good friends, and we went hiking where there were ginger flowers growing along the trails. This was a positive association with a very happy time of my life, when I was exploring this very vibrant and alive jungle environment, doing a lot of athletic and energetic climbing. At a time when I was in a hospital bed I had this memory association with exercise and the reddish purple ginger flowers of New Guinea. It was a very strong, positive feeling.

Angela Peroba

A reporter in her thirties
Salvador, Bahia, Brazil

Kendra: Angela had been trying to conceive a child for a
number of years, and she and her husband had already
done several different tests and treatments. It was discovered that she had a small obstruction in one of her fallop-
ian tubes, but this was not a probable reason for her
inability to conceive. She was seeing a psychotherapist at
the time I saw her and she was eager to try everything
available that may have a chance of helping her. I spoke
to her about psycho-aromatherapy and she wanted to try
aromas. We scheduled an appointment and I brought a
calming oil with me, the absolute of orange blossom.
First we had a conversation, and she told me in detail the
situation and her issues with this problem. Soon I noticed
that she was trying to help her body with her mind, but
as she went with more and more concepts, she would
churn and churn large amounts of stress-forming material. I knew this session had to be with body and scent and
leaving the mind with just the decision of the image she

needed to associate to the smell of orange blossoms, to benefit her. I gave her a full body massage, with the intent of our decision in mutual focus. It was pretty obvious to me as I started that the problem in her body was fear-based tension developed to such an extent that her reproductive function was shutting down. If only she could get herself to relax, she would conceive. I left her with an aromatic crystal, some more neroli oil, and a massage oil with the same aroma in more diluted form for her to use daily on her abdomen and use to do a little meditation keeping the focus of what we had registered at the time of the therapy. After our treatment she felt very optimistic and continued searching for more help from metaphysical, spiritual, and traditional medical methods. Less than two months later, already in the States, I received a letter from her, giving me the happy news of her first pregnancy.

Angela: I feel something opened with our aroma work. I thank you again. I feel from this experience with aromatherapy that it is somehow difficult to separate what happened in my body, emotions, and mind. When I reflect on it, what becomes clear is that this therapy via aroma worked in me in a very effective way that I want to call global. Principally, it provided me a trust that my searching was going to succeed. With the orange blossom, I felt my trust growing as if I was being showered with the scent of happiness. Next to the trust, I felt a synchronicity with more serenity between my internal and external movements. Without a doubt, the aromatherapy participated electively and in a holistic way with the traditional medicine that I engaged in shortly afterwards.

One thing that becomes ever so obvious to me is that these therapies all have a common denominator—they help an individual to focus on creating a change, or making their experience of self more coherent in a holistic way. Each person also became more aware of their emotions, their environment, and of others around them. This helps them to create a positive change in their condition. These are broad aspects. There are also many nuances that become clear once one is engaged in these therapies. Substance addiction, child abuse, autism, terminal patients and the dying, childbirth and other conditions are greatly benefitted by therapies using aroma, especially with flower oils, which generally have a good acceptance.

Following are a few facts concerning the sense of smell:

The act of smelling will stimulate alertness, memory and learning, sensitivity, self-esteem, awareness of wholeness, receptivity to information, elimination of stress, and reproductive system functions.

Sexual excitement increases olfactory capacity.

Olfactory deprivation can contribute to Alzheimer's disease and madness.

Sensory deprivation can mutate genetic codes.

A child and mother can identify each other solely by smell.

One may not be able to relax in an environment with unfamiliar smells.

The smell of body odors are affected by diet.

Stress, habitual stressful thoughts, and other emotional conditions modify body odor.

Part of male and female attraction is processed via smell.

Pheromones—chemicals detected in sweat, urine, and feces—also exist in the vomenal nasal organ and are molecules containing messages that trigger sexual behavior.

Smell being processed by the right brain stimulates the feeling center.

Body Odor Meditation

This is an exercise that will heighten your awareness of self and stimulate conscious holistic self-learning and acceptance, to give you a sense of internal harmony and peace. To do it, you need to be ready for a lesson of surrender, humility, facing fear, and concentration. This meditation is done in a bathtub in a silent and dim environment, and you will need to have a natural sweaty body with the absence of any body care products. You can do it after a busy working day, after working out, or after a couple of days without bathing.

Center yourself and calm your thinking process. Direct focus on yourself and your breathing pattern. Fill the bathtub with water as hot as you can tolerate. If it is winter, make sure the bathroom is warm. Slowly place yourself in the water to cover only up to your waist. Sit comfortably and soon you should begin to sweat notice-ably. Concentrate on the perception of positive feelings you have had about yourself. Take time with yourself, emptying your mind and just feeling your body and emotions. Soon you will begin to feel surrounded by your own body smell. Focus on placing no judgment and relax into it in equanimity. Develop the situation to the point that you are breathing freely and enjoyably, with the focus of your own body odor surrounding you. When you feel that you have experienced the totality of this encounter with self, you can bathe and get out of the experience. Notice what happens in your relationship with yourself in the days that follow this experience.

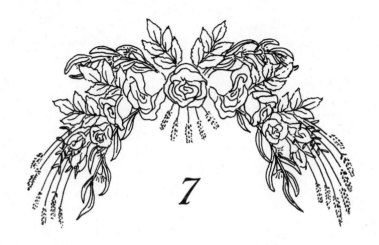

7

The Use of Scent in Magic

The Tangibility of the Invisible

*M*agic uses intention and power or will to believe in one's own ability to create out of nothing and combine elements to successfully emit concepts and energy that can have a tangible effect. I believe magic is real because one can feel it. Feelings are very real. One can also observe magic; you can witness your own transformation and that of others while you apply magic to an organism, object, or place.

Magic is the art of meeting, surrounding, emitting, and extracting—to perform transformation and change of consciousness in the mind or the physical world. In doing magic, one has to become aware of the physical and the non-physical at the same time and focus on that union.

Let's take the aroma of an essential oil. The essential oil is physical and tangible. The element of imagination that you use in your magic is non-physical and intangible, but the aroma of your essential oil is very tangible because you can smell it. The smell is physical because it consists of aromatic molecules in spite of being invisible to the naked eye.

Essential oils can teach you how to work with the invisible if you begin to perceive the aromatic molecules as energy that transforms you in the same way that the invisible energies flowing through the magic you create can also make you more calm or energized. You can use an essential oil to bring your magic into a more tangible form. This is because the invisible but tangible element of the essential oils—the smell—will serve as a bridge between the intangible reality of invisible energies, which can be felt but not touched, and the ordinary palpable reality that is physical.

The aromatic energy of the essence is very volatile; it escapes the physical world very quickly and goes elsewhere. Where does it go? It certainly goes to your mind, and mingles with memory and emotion. But it also goes to the environment. Does it do to the environment what it does to your mind? What does it do to your mind? I have just stated that it can have a calming or exciting effect, for instance, or it can trigger all kinds of complex feelings having to do with what was in your memory bank and your imagination. Essential oil molecules, because of their smell, easily merge with the images you visualize, creating a dynamic living field of energy. So if visualization has always been an important element in magic, imagine how much more powerful it becomes in combination with an aroma. You can use the field of energy created by images and aromatic molecules to emit messages or to surround someone—maybe an emotionally disturbed person—during therapy.

What about the environment? Is there connected to it a parallel dimension as intangible as your imagination and as tangible as your invisible aroma, one that relates to your body and mind in the same way that it relates to the rest of nature?

I can only tell you that I know this to be true, and that the energy that lives there is also affected by your aromatic essence, as well as by other invisible elements that you can feel and use in your magic.

Now imagine that some of that energy from our parallel dimension is the energy of nature spirits, elementals, fairies, or whatever else you want to call it, that relates to plant life. Consider that this energy only takes form when it meets the imagination that can design concepts for their form, simple or complex.

Let's call this image a symbol. It has form and information about its function. Symbols have the ability to expand into information. Information communicates through light, that medium that travels through all dimensions—physical and non-physical.

The work of gathering symbols to be used in magic is the work of creating a graphic notion for that which you have experienced and learned in your life and that has enough meaning for you to use. For example, if you once felt very stressed and confused and decided to retreat alone in nature to relax, and there you felt the powerful presence of the earth giving you strength to cope and modify your condition, you discover an equation you can use: *earth = strength*. You can condense this experience into a symbol—maybe it can be just a shell or a rock you picked up, or a simple shape you glimpsed on a leaf at the very moment of your realization, and that stayed in your mind. You can use this symbol in your magic to recall the emotion of that experience, to be used at the appropriate time and for the appropriate reason. If you combine this symbol with a scent, then you will expand your ability to recall the experience with great power.

Once you have created a symbol—or collected symbols containing personal information—and you want to use them, you must coordinate them into usable form by creating a special place where you can focus and use as a point of reference. Next, with love, invoke the invisible energies and open yourself to intuition and to the light to bring you insight. Continuing, use your breath, the scent you chose, movement, sound, or whatever is your resource and inspiration at the time. Depending on what your intention and will is, the movement of energy in your magical act of power will vary in direction. Perhaps you will call a meeting with another field of energy, or maybe you are sending a telepathic message, correcting imbalances in a body, or surrounding a place with peace.

After I am finished with magical acts of power, I always remember to disassemble and release into the earth all energies invoked and gathered. I find this process useful in order to seal the transformation from my experience within, so that it naturally integrates into my ordinary reality without the risk of becoming dogmatic with the form of the magical space I created. I only understand that one should keep a physical space of magical symbols in the case of devotional practice when one is able and willing to tend to it on a continuous basis.

Now let's leave the logical mind for a moment and step into the right brain functions for a simple and wonderful exercise of aroma magic.

Imagine a field full of lavender flowers. If you already know lavender flowers or the oil, your mind can invoke a memory for it. Or you can choose a different oil or aromatic plant that you know.

Now imagine that energy (that you can smell) in your mind as a very impressionable energy, like a photographic plate. Now use visualization, one of your magical elements, and slowly design a form for what we will call the spirit of lavender flowers. Imagine and feel that energy from the field of flowers taking the form of your design and creating an image. This image will always be saved in your memory bank . . . aaahhh . . . now STOP. Notice how you feel. Quickly write two words to describe how you feel. Did anything change in your being since you started this exercise? Now take a bottle of lavender, pour a drop on a cloth, and inhale. Take a few inhalations and repeat the exercise. Hold on to your image and the feeling. Notice and write down how you feel. These feelings come from the interaction with the spirit of lavender.

If you take the inspirations from this exercise further, it will give you insightful information and a bond will be created between you and the lavender. You will feel that you know it better and you will feel the dynamics of its energy in a playful way. This interaction can lead to more magic, which can develop as a style to get to know an essential oil.

In co-creating with the invisible energy of the oils, holding a clear intention and carrying a bond for further interactions, subliminally you will be receiving information from the codes in the molecules themselves, which all proceed from the greater living organism, the earth. Let your imagination take form in myriad combinations and explore with many essences in this way. This has always helped me in my blending and perfume making.

Aroma magic will always be as powerful and real to me as unconditional love.

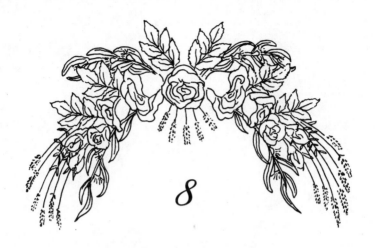

8

Vibrational Medicine

Essential Oil Synergies

*A*s we become one with our natural environment, we begin to understand it. By entraining ourselves with different elements of nature, be it a natural stone, a plant essence, the sound of the wind on a tree branch, or the sight of the sunset colors, we can create a synergy by using our biological systems and program information using intention, to bring ourselves to a state of harmony and health.

This is a natural and holistic science that vibrational medicine understands. Vibrational medicine is a new system of thinking about healing that recognizes the body's many unified fields of energy and how they are interconnected.

I look at a healing practice as a creative endeavor, an art in which a lot of joy can move freely during the focus on love energy. I have witnessed wonderful results with this, playing with crystals, natural colored stones, essential oils, and the sounds that we can vibrate using our vocal cords. This brings to the body energies that can affect the coherent function of our unified fields of energy. When our different fields align and merge, we are uplifted and growth in our states of consciousness results from the created harmony. This is the kind of therapy that can be of use with cancer and AIDS patients, as well as in the common stress-related conditions. What I love about this type of healing is that it is free from labeling or direction from techniques that are the workings of the logical thinking mind. It relies mainly on feeling, intuitive knowing, and love. Techniques are a product of the logical mind and are limited, not free from concept-dependent risks of the personality centered perceptions. Individual systems are often too specialized and without accurate self-knowledge. As the late scientist Marcel Vogel, Ph.D., of the Psychic Research Institute in San Jose, California, would put it, *love is full spectrum energy.* Love comes from a total system, rather than a partial one. This way we are sure to be covering the totality of a field.

Facts About Quartz Crystals

It is important to mention some of the results that Marcel Vogel, found in his work with liquid crystals. He was able to determine in his lab, through various measurements using spectrographic analysis, that we can create change in matter with our thoughts. Our thoughts create measurable vibrations that can have an influence in matter such as water, stones, our bodies, and other biological systems.

Vogel used crystals as a means to transfer thoughts to water and was able to measure changes in aluminum conductivity, surface tension, ultraviolet frequencies, and the like. Liquid crystal, which we have in our bodies, is a state between a solid and a liquid. Liquid crystals, are equal to quartz crystals, in that they are highly organized chemical structures that can reproduce themselves and transfer information between molecules through photonic emission or light—electromagnetic radiation.

Liquid crystals communicate information between our cells within our biological systems. Quartz crystal can receive the vibratory information from thoughts into its geometric chemical lattice structure and communicate it to another unified field of energy. The concept is very much like a computer function where you have an image, the icon representing the stored information that one can drag with the mouse to another application. Thus, information can be carried out in an efficient way without loss of energy.

We are discovering that the key to biological systems lies in being able to transfer information and self-replicate. When it can replicate itself, it can continue on with the record and communicate the information.

Besides this ability, we also know that quartz crystals have physical properties of piezoeletricity, which means that quartz crystals emit an electric charge if stimulated mechanically, and conversely quartz crystal will oscillate in a constant rhythm if an electric current is put into it. This is currently largely explored in telecommunications and remote sensing technology.

The Spiral

The universal consciousness thinks in mathematical codes perhaps to be able to record, amplify and transmit energy, and manipulate matter. In nature there are geometric patterns that repeat themselves in a certain proportional aspect. This situation has been referred to as "the golden rule." The golden rule defines this harmonious aspect found in nature with evidence creating the understanding of the proportions and patterns that repeat themselves over and over again in such natural elements as flowers, crystals, and snowflakes. (For more information, refer to *The Power of Limits* by Gyorgy Doczi.) There is a constant element that we observe to be always present, which is the spiraling effect. This is present in the chemical structure of quartz crystals and also in our DNA, giving us a clue that must point to great synchronicity and synergy potential between these two energy fields.

Intention

As quartz crystals have the ability to store information, it is important to have a clear focus and great awareness of intention when handling them so that what it is helping you manifest in your life is what you want. I always use a powerful forced exhale with the intention of clearing a crystal, deleting all psychic energies that may be contained in it, and use another exhalation to program a given intention. This is probably as far as I go with techniques. Sometimes, I simply look at a crystal with the intention to will it clean of unwanted vibrations, or leave crystals to interact with the element: in the rain, into the earth, safely in a stream bed, or under the sunshine or moonshine.

Natural Colored Stones: Color and Light

Natural colored stones, as well as colorless stones such as quartz and diamond, are physical forms containing the highest rate of vibrations from the mineral kingdom. As each color in the spectrum is a specification of light, one could perceive natural stones as frozen light. Through light we receive information. An ordinary way to explain this is with an analogy of a dark room. In a dark room we have no idea of the colors or shapes of objects in it. As soon as we turn on the light, we see it all almost instantaneously. The interaction with a stone provides us vast amounts of information on numerous levels of our perception, conscious and unconscious. This process is extremely individual because each person operates at a different level of sensitivity.

Trace metal elements in the crystal structure and their interaction with light makes the color of a stone. There is spectro-transmission and spectro-absorption to create the color of a stone. Full spectro-transmission means that all the light is being transmitted through the stone. Full spectro-absorption means that all the light that is moving through the stone is being absorbed by the stone. These are the black stones, such as black jade or black tourmaline.

The color of a stone depends on the vibratory rate at which a stone absorbs the light. For example, ruby is red, indicating that the only part of the spectrum that is being transmitted from the stone is the red ray of the spectrum. All the other rates of the spectrum—the greens and the blues, et cetera—are being captured by the stone. So a stone is really serving the specialized purpose of directing that ray of the light to the surrounding environment. The light goes in and vibrates in the stone. The stone is at a certain frequency due to its chemical composition and structure. The light that comes out is the reflection of the frequency of the light that is being transmitted. If the red part of the spectrum is what is being held in the stone—which is a slower vibration than the greens, blues, and violets—then what is going to be transmitted is a color at a higher frequency than the red, which could be a green, or another higher frequency color depending on the chemical composition and frequency rate of the stone. This is only mentioning the colors that are perceived by the naked eye, without going into the ultraviolets or infrareds, which our vision does not perceive.

Colorless stones like quartz and diamond are transmitting all the frequency rates of the spectrum—all colors—so they are like the light itself in a general sense. These colorless stones can create a prismatic effect. The light that is speeding through the atmosphere hits the solid matter of a colorless stone body at an angle and slows down as it penetrates the crystal, which bends the light. It is this bending of the light that creates a separation of the spectrum and creates the prismatic rainbow that we see. The colors all have different rates of vibration and different speeds. This is how the colors separate, because they are vibrating at different rates as the light penetrates the crystal. Lower frequencies are slower, higher frequencies are faster. The order from slower to faster is red, yellow, green, blue, indigo, and violet.

The Nutro-Vibrational Chain

Minerals break down into soil and release all their elements. Plants take these elements into their bodies and combine them with metals that were once rocks into a system with organic molecules. We eat the plants and absorb the metals and trace elements that are so important in the biological functions of our bodies. This cycle, which illustrates so well how everything is connected, I call the nutro-vibrational chain. As we receive the nourishment from the elements ingested, we also receive the informational codes that are vibrational and are being transmitted throughout all the kingdoms of nature, uniting and connecting us to the full cycle that is the continuous movement of life. When we die, all the elements or elementals that were invested into our unified field of energy go back to the energy field of the matrix, the earth, going through all the kingdoms again.

Synergy of Natural Stones with Essential Oils

Crystals and natural colored stones or gems have the highest frequency of the mineral kingdom. Likewise, essential oils are the distilled elixir of highest vibrations from the plant kingdom—the volatile, the spirit of the plant. When we humans synergize these two powers and apply the result to our energy fields, a strong influence from the highest earth frequency is created in our electromagnetic circuitry.

It is impossible not to be affected with all kinds of magnetic information and light emissions. But why do we do these things? I think we are living in an era when we are very active in our will to become aware of much more than we have been, both in ourselves and with the environment. These new experiences create more possibilities for us, and it all has to do with the perception of the invisible vibrational realities, which we begin to know when we become more aware and sensitive to ourselves and our environment.

At this point, I share with you my experience of creating my line of aromatic stones and jewelry known as Aromajewels.

Kendra's Aromajewels

My first thought about creating Aromajewels held an ancient feeling, almost as if I was hearing whispers of the past coming from the future. It had that timeless quality and the experience of harmonious wonder that I often feel when I am working with stones and with essential oils, but putting the two together in a synergy really lifted me to an exalted state of consciousness, something like riding on a forever flying magic carpet. It is difficult to explain this feeling. Words fail to describe the enormous pleasure of experiencing such stones on my body and energy field.

All the time I spent with my first Aromajewels, I could feel nature—the elementals of plant and mineral—working with me, and I became accustomed to receiving information from their fields, feeling that the human element of thought and intention manifested as the design and manufacture that I provided to make this entity a physical reality was a source of joy in the other dimensions involved. Together we were perceiving the workings of a fabulous synergy! The Aromajewel was better than the essential oil in the bottle, it was better than the rough piece of stone, and it was better than my thoughts, drawings, and wax models. Together we did it! We created a synergy of the best natural elements from the mineral and plant kingdoms as a gift to the human world.

Aromajewels themselves are more dynamic than a glass container, and they serve a function of communicating the life and properties of the essential oils, magnified through the crystal, directly to the electromagnetic field of the body. This transmits a high frequency impact, which affects the different energy fields, causing them to merge and harmonize. With a programmed intention and the knowledge of the synergies and their function, you can create a specific healing practice. In this, there is the addition of our human consciousness and full spectrum love energy to make it even more powerful and global (see chart on page 227). This work with the jewels can become specialized to be applied in healing, and there are a prolific number of synergetic possibilities and their functions. For instance, a certain stone, with its vibratory rate emitting a certain ray of the spectrum—let's say blue in an aquamarine, which has been experienced as a calming, relaxing influence—can be combined with an essential oil that emits this same vibratory rate, let's say blue chamomile.

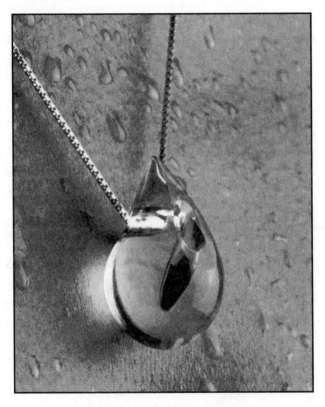

*An Aromajewel aromatic quartz crystal
drop pendant with blue chamomile.*

The fairly high rates of vibration of the color blue in the oil and from the stone can be combined with a fairly high pitch of a sound vibrating from our vocal cords. This brings the energy fields into coherence with a very powerful calming effect.

By common sense, it is important to note here that the color of an oil is not the only factor to determine its frequency, as is the case with natural stones. The essential oil is derived from the plant, so it is more accurate to determine its frequency by analyzing the plant that the oil came from, taking into consideration the possible manifested colors in the plant, such as the flowers or other parts.

We did a two-day research experiment with kirlian photography using an aromatic crystal and different essential oils with calming and energizing actions to see if we could obtain a graphic representation of change in the electromagnetic field. We used the Biofeedback Imaging Color Spectrometer 3000, a photographic unit consisting of high speed imaging, high voltage integrated with biofeedback technology. After photographing before and after shots of six different people with different essential oils in a quartz crystal pendant, we noticed what seemed to be a common denominator: the blocks of color that appeared in all the "before" images always become homogeneous and more vibrant in the second image, after the aromatic crystal pendant had been placed on the thymus area of the user. This happened whether the essential oil was calming or energizing. My own conclusion is that what I saw was a graphic representation of the influence of harmonization, alignment, or coherence in the user's energy field caused by the effect of the essential oils and the quartz crystal. I believe we may have just touched on something that we may take to further, more complex experiments, to be able to graphically prove the action of these different natural elements in the electromagnetic field.

Sound

Sound has been documented as influencing biological functions in the body that affect all cells, causing measurable biological function changes. Sound stimulates all the senses through entrainment, a vibratory response creating synchronicity between fields. When sound is used at the same time that the color vibration from a stone and an oil is used—which are both transmitting electromagnetic emissions to a field—this powerful influence creates efficient therapeutics for sedating somebody's agitated field, for example. There are numerous possibilities, even considering only the visible color spectrum and the different sounds in toning with the notes of the musical scale in variations of all the vowels. For these enjoyable possibilities see the chart on page 227 for suggested combinations.

Chakras

The chakras are the gateways from and to the different consciousness levels of our unified fields of energy. The chakras move according to different vibratory rates, like the musical scale and the color spectrum going from the lowest frequency rate to the highest. This can be easily correlated to all the other aspects manifested with a frequency rate scale, especially colors. The chakras correspond to the nervous system network and the endocrine glands. They receive information from more subtle fields of energy within the same system and transfer this energy to the physical body through the nervous system and the endocrine glands, and consequently to the organs of the body.

Profiles of Natural Stones

Following is a list of a selection of stones, in the order of the visible color spectrum, that are the most accessible in stores all over the world. The information contained in this session was derived from learning about rocks with Brian Cook, the mineral books in the appendix, and my own knowledge from studying and working with rocks since the 1970s. Note that the scale of hardness of stones is from 1 to 10. Diamond is 10, our teeth rate a 5. Definition of piezoelectric properties occurs earlier in this chapter, on page 196.

Purple Quartz-Amythyst

Chemical family: Silicates.

System: Rhombohedral-hexagonal.

Composition: Silica and oxygen, with trace amounts of ferric iron, which colors it violet.

Place of origin: Brazil, Uruguay, Sri Lanka, Canada, Russia, United States, and Africa.

Characteristics: Usually occurs in well-formed crystals, more common in clusters or geodes. Transparent to translucent. Hardness of 7. Piezoelectric properties.

Color: Varies from lavender to deep purple.

History and lore: Purple quartz has been used since early times as a cure for drunkenness and uncontrollable love passion. Influenced by Mars and Jupiter.

Astrological sign: Pisces.

Therapeutic and metaphysical information: Stimulates memory, enhancing mental functions. Remedy for insomnia and headaches. Transmutation of energy, purification, ascension. The stone of Saint Germain and the seventh ray.

Blue Corundum-Sapphire

Chemical family: Oxides.

System: Hexagonal.

Composition: Oxygen, hydrogen, and aluminum.

Place of origin: Africa, Burma, India, Sri Lanka, Thailand, and the United States.

Characteristics: One of the hardest translucent gemstones, with a hardness of 9. Found as well-formed crystals or stream gravels.

Color: Corundum is also ruby, which occurs blood red. Corundum also occurs in green, pink, orange, yellow, and purple. Blue sapphire varies in hue, reaching a desirable vibration of indigo blue. Most commercial stones have been heated to obtain a higher quality blue.

History and lore: In old England, blue sapphire was used in the treatment of the contagious diseases of the eyes. Ruled by planets Jupiter and Mercury.

Therapeutic and metaphysical information: Blue sapphire is used to treat mental illnesses, rheumatism, and intestinal disorders in Ayurvedic medicine. Relates to the throat chakra and the pituitary gland. Stimulant of the functions related to the solar plexus.

Blue Beryl-Aquamarine

Chemical family: Silicates.

System: Hexagonal.

Composition: Beryllium, aluminum, silica.

Place of origin: Afghanistan, Brazil, Italy, Nigeria, United States, and Russia.

Characteristics: Very hard, 7.5 to 8. Translucent. Occurs with well-formed crystals.

Color: Blue of a light hue going to a maximum medium blue.

History and lore: Used by high priests in the first century B.C. *Aquamarine* means "sea water." Ruled by the planet Venus.

Therapeutic and metaphysical information: Relates to treating inflammation of the eyes and swollen glands, especially in throat area. Assists in emotional stability and clear communication, cleanser of the throat chakra. Yin influence.

Green Tourmaline

Chemical family: Silicates.

System: Trigonal.

Composition: Complex borosilicates containing magnesium, iron, aluminum, manganese, lithium, silica, or oxygen.

Place of origin: Africa, Brazil, Italy, United States, and Russia.

Characteristics: Hardness of 7.5 to 8. Translucent. Piezoelectric properties. Well-formed crystals. Complex mineral occurring in all colors of the spectrum.

Color: Green tourmaline varies from light butter lettuce green to a deep, almost black green.

History and lore: A stone exploited in recent history, after the discovery of the new world, in Brazil. Explorers were looking for emeralds and thought they had found emerald mines when they discovered green tourmalines. Ruled by the planet Pluto.

Therapeutic properties and metaphysical information: Immune system and cardiac strengthener. Green tourmaline relates to the herbs that have affinity with healing heart conditions.

Green Beryl-Emerald

Chemical family: Silicates.

System: Hexagonal.

Composition: Beryllium aluminum silicate.

Place of origin: Afghanistan, Africa, Brazil, Colombia, and the United States.

Characteristics: Very hard but brittle, 7.5 to 8. Transparent, well-formed crystals.

Color: Light to dark green.

History and lore: Attributed to having a prophetic quality of showing the future through visions seen in the stone. Used for checking the truth in others. Ruled by Venus and Mercury.

Therapeutic properties and metaphysical information:
Valuable for strengthening the spinal column. Stone of general healing energies dealing with issues of manifesting truth. Relates to the heart chakra. Balanced between Yin and Yang.

Yellow Quartz-Citrine

Chemical family: Silicates.

System: Rhombohedral-Hexagonal.

Composition: Oxygen, silica, and iron hydrates.

Place of origin: Brazil, France, Madagascar, and Russia.

Characteristics: Hardness of 7. Piezoelectric properties. Transparent and sometimes occurring as well-formed crystals.

Color: Varies from a clear ivory yellow to a yellow, a smoky yellow, and a rare rich amber gold.

Therapeutic properties and metaphysical information:
Healing influence for those suffering from asthma. This is a yang vibrational influence for the solar plexus helping

disperse blocking energies from negative emotions that are keeping the body in a morbid state.

Rutilated Quartz

Chemical family: Quartz: Silicates. Rutile: Oxides.

System: Quartz: Rhombohedral-Hexagonal. Rutile: Tetragonal.

Composition: Quartz: Oxygen and silica. Rutile: Oxygen, Titanium.

Place of origin: Brazil, Madagascar, and Switzerland.

Characteristics: Well-formed quartz crystals containing rutile crystals captured inside its structure. Hardness of 7 for the quartz and 6 to 6.5 for the rutile crystals. Piezoelectric properties.

Color: Quartz can be clear or smoky. The smoky color is caused by exposure to natural radioactivity. The rutile crystals can occur in different hues of gold, copper, reddish, or silvery color.

History and lore: Not existent in records to my knowledge.

Therapeutic and metaphysical information: I have been living with abundant rutilated quartz in my environment for sixteen years, and I have distinctly observed that is has an energizing effect on the nervous system and the solar plexus. Balanced between yin and yang.

Gurudas writes that rutilated quartz "helps assimilation of life force, and all nutrients are easier assimilated. Tends to reverse disorders associated with a lowered immune system." It helps to speed up the information passing between neurons.

Orange Topaz-Imperial

Chemical family: Silicates.

System: Orthorhombic.

Composition: Aluminum, iron, hydrogen, oxygen, and silica.

Place of origin: Brazil and Siberia.

Characteristics: Very hard, but brittle, hardness of 8. Translucent, bright luster. Occurs as well-formed crystals.

Color: Light, medium, and deep golden orange and pinkish orange.

History and lore: This stone has a curious lore of being looked at by seamen for guidance during nights with no moon to guide their course. Seen as having affinity with the light of the sun, it was used to assuage fear of the night.

Therapeutic and metaphysical information: Relates to all conditions requiring vitality, warmth, and yang energy. Rejuvenation. Dynamic living symbol for divine love. Ruled by the sun and Saturn, relates to the solar plexus. Yang.

Rose Quartz

Chemical family: Silicates.

System: Hexagonal.

Composition: Oxygen, silica, manganese, titanium.

Place of origin: Brazil, Madagascar, and United States.

Characteristics: Hardness of 7. Piezoelectric properties.

Translucent. Rarely occurs as well-formed crystals, more commonly found in masses. Often included and fractured.

Color: Varies from a clear light to medium pink and milky baby pink.

History and lore: This stone has no recorded history to my knowledge.

Therapeutic and metaphysical information: Relates to feelings and the heart with a tranquilizing effect. It is helpful to balance emotions affecting internal organs. Balance between yin and yang, ruled by planet Venus.

Garnet-Red

Chemical family: Silicates.

System: Isometric.

Composition: Aluminum, calcium magnesium, oxygen, silica.

Place of origin: Brazil, Czechoslovakia, India, United States, Siberia, and Africa.

Characteristics: Hardness between 6.5 and 7.5. Translucent to transparent. Well-formed gyrodal crystals.

Color: Varies in all the hues of oranges, reds, and reddish browns.

History and lore: Sacred stone to the Native American Indians, Aztecs, and other native peoples throughout the world. It was also used in the breastplates of high priests in the Middle Ages. It was used as protection against the spilling of blood in wars.

Therapeutic and metaphysical properties: Red garnet relates to the sacral chakra as a purifying and invigorating influence. Circulatory conditions and sexual ailments; energies of manifestation and strong movement of energy.

Red Tourmaline

Chemical family: Silicates.

Composition: Complex borosilicates containing magnesium, iron, aluminum, manganese, lithium, silica, or oxygen.

Place of Origin: Afghanistan, Brazil, Madagascar, and the United States.

Characteristics: Hardness of 7.5. Transparent to translucent.

Piezoelectric properties. Well-formed crystals known as rubellite.

Color: Varies from lovely violet pink, to pink-pink and deep red.

Therapeutic and metaphysical uses: Relates to stimulating circulatory movement of the blood and frequencies merging the sexual with the heart chakra vibrations. Relates to the sacral chakra. Yang.

Quartz-Smoky

Chemical family: Silicates.

System: Rhombohedral-Hexagonal.

Composition: Silica and oxygen.

Place of origin: Brazil, Scotland, Switzerland, United States.

Characteristics: Occurs as well-formed crystals and in uncrystallized masses. Transparent. Hardness of 7. Piezoelectric properties. The smoky color is caused by exposure to natural radioactivity.

Color: Varies from gray to amber brown and deep brown.

Therapeutic and metaphysical information: Maintains quality of grounding static energies from all the chakras, balanced yin and yang polarities. Relates to the base chakra. Introspection.

Black Tourmaline

Chemical family: Silicates.

System: Trigonal.

Composition: Complex borosilicates containing magnesium, iron, aluminum, manganese, lithium, silica, or oxygen.

Place of origin: Brazil and the United States.

Characteristics: Hardness of 7.5. Piezoelectric properties. Well-formed crystals.

Color: Opaque black with highly lustrous surface.

Therapeutic and metaphysical information: Used for treating those exposed to radiation. Highly absorbent quality, checking out negative energies.

Black Jade

Chemical family: Silicates.

System: Monoclynic.

Composition: Aluminum, iron, silica, and sodium.

Place of Origin: Australia, Burma, China, and United States.

Characteristics: Hardness of 6.5 to 7, crystallized form very rare. Compact and tough. Opaque to translucent. Partially translucent.

Color: Jadeite occurs in all colors including black and white.

History and lore: Considered a sacred stone to different native tribes of the world. Used on the breastplate of the medieval high priest. Chinese cultures hold jade in high esteem relating it to longevity, male fertility, and kidney-related disorders.

Therapeutic and metaphysical information: A stone of endurance, integrity, and equanimity, effecting vibrational influences to all conditions requiring these qualities. Base chakra.

Diamond

Chemical family: Native element.

System: Isometric.

Composition: Carbon.

Place of origin: Australia, Brazil, Africa, the United States, and numerous other countries all over the world.

Characteristics: Hardest mineral on earth, 10. Beautiful octahedron crystals, transparent with high surface luster.

Color: Colorless but also occurring in translucent hues of yellow, blue, green, gray, peach, brown, and black.

History and lore: Regarded as a symbol for invulnerability, the diamond has an extensive history of being ingested for all kinds of purposes and ailments, from removing kidney stones to providing superior strength and good luck. Used as jewelry by medieval high priests. Ruled by Venus and Jupiter. Balance between yin and yang.

Therapeutic and metaphysical information: Manifestation of the perfect balance between energy and matter, it transmits the full spectrum of colors and the totality of light frequencies. It can be used in synergy with all other stones, further empowering their specific ray transmission, and it can improve or extend the qualities of a stone where the quality is not optimum. Like the quartz crystal, the diamond can be used in every way with all synergies, but it carries a warmer energy than the quartz, which is cooling.

Clear Quartz

Chemical family: Silicates.

System: Rhombohedron-Hexagonal.

Composition: Silica and oxygen.

Place of origin: All over the world.

Characteristics: Occurs as well-formed crystals and in uncrystallized masses. Transparent to translucent. Hardness of 7. Piezoelectric properties.

Color: Colorless.

History and lore: Used as a sacred object by shamans of many native peoples all over the world. Relates to the element silver and to the moon.

Therapeutic and metaphysical information: Like the diamond, clear quartz transmits the full spectrum and can be used in any synergy. Mainly used as a transducer and recorder of energy. Please refer to page 195 for facts about quartz.

Vibrational Medicine
Chakra Correspondences

Chakra	Color	Stone	Essential Oil	Sound	Body System or Organ
base	black, brown, red	black tourmaline, black jade, garnet, red tourmaline, smoky quartz	frankincense, myrrh, patchuli, vetiver	toning of all vowels in DO	blood circulation, gonads
sacral	red, orange,	garnet, imperial topaz, red tourmaline, rose quartz	jasmine, rose, sandalwood, ylang-ylang	toning of all vowels in RE	sexual organs, urinary system
solar plexus	yellow, gold	citrine, rutilated quartz, golden beryl	basil, clary sage, lemon, orange blossom	toning of all vowels in MI	digestive system, stomach, liver, adrenal glands
heart	green, pink	emerald, green tourmaline, pink tourmaline, rose quartz	bergamot, geranium, orange blossom, rose	toning of all vowels in FA	circulatory system, heart, thymus gland

continued

Chakra	Color	Stone	Essential Oil	Sound	Body System or Organ
throat	light and medium blue, silver	aquamarine, blue tourmaline, silver	all chamomiles, orange blossom (neroli)	toning of all vowels in SOL	respiratory system, lungs, thyroid gland
third eye	lavender, deep blue, indigo	deep blue tourmalines, sapphire, amethyst	lavender, rosemary	toning of all vowels in LA	nervous system, pituitary gland
crown	violet, gold, white	amethyst, diamond, gold	frankincense, jasmine, lavender, sandalwood	toning of all vowels in SI and high DO	central nervous system, pineal gland

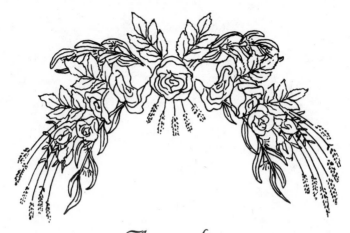

Appendix

Aromatherapy Resources

Suggested Reading

Aromatherapy, Essential Oils and Other Related Work

Berwick, Ann. *Holistic Aromatherapy: Balance the Body and Soul with Essential Oils.* St. Paul, MN: Llewellyn Publications, 1994.

Cunningham, Scott. *Magical Aromatherapy.* St. Paul, MN: Llewellyn Publications, 1989.

Damian, Peter and Kate. *Aromatherapy: Scent and Psyche.* New York: Inner Traditions, 1995.

Davis, Patricia. *Aromatherapy: An A to Z.* Saffron Walden, England: C. W. Daniel, 1988.

———. *Subtle Aromatherapy.* Saffron Walden, England: C. W. Daniel, 1991.

England, Allison. *Aromatherapy for Mother and Baby.* Rochester, VT: Healing Arts Press, 1994.

Fawcett, Margaret, R. M. *Aromatherapy for Pregnancy and Childbirth.* New York: Penguin, 1993.

Franchomme, P. and D. Pénoël. *L'aromatherapie exactment.* Roger Jollois, 1990.

Gattefosse, Rene-Maurice. *Gattefosse's Aromatherapy.* Saffron Walden, England: C. W. Daniel, 1993.

Green, Minday and Katty Keville. *Aromatherapy: A Complete Guide to the Healing Art.* Freedom, CA: Crossing Press, 1995.

Lawless, Julia. *"Illustraded" Encyclopedia of Essential Oils.* Revised Edition. Shaftesbury, Dorset: Element, 1995.

———. *Aromatherapy and the Mind.* New York: Harper Collins.

Lavabre, Marcel. *Aromatherapy Workbook.* Rochester, VT: Healing Arts Press, 1990.

Lawless, Julia. *The Encyclopedia of Essential Oils.* Shaftesbury, Dorset: Element, 1992.

Maury, M. Marguerite. *Maury's Guide to Aromatherapy.* Saffron Walden, England: C. W. Daniel, 1988.

Miller, Light and Bryan. *Ayurveda and Aromatherapy.* Lotus Light, 1996.

Price, Shirley. *Practical Aromatherapy.* Wellingborough, England: Thorsons, 1983.

———. *Aromatherapy for Health Professionals.* New York: Churchill Livingston, 1995.

Rose, Jeanne. *The Aromatherapy Book.* Berkeley, CA: North Atlantic Books, 1992.

Rose Jeanne, Eartl and Susan, eds. *The World of Aromatherapy.* Clarksdale, MS: Frog Ltd., 1996.

Schnaubelt, Kurt, Ph.D. *Advanced Aromatherapy.* Virginia Beach, VA: Inner Visions, 1997.

Scholes, M. *Pocket Guide to Aromatherapy.* Aromatherapy Seminars, 1993.

Tisserand, Maggie. *Aromatherapy for Women.* Wellingborough, England: Thorsons, 1985.

Tisserand, Robert. *The Art of Aromatherapy.* New York: Inner Traditions, 1977.

————. *The E.O. Safety Data Manual.* Tisserand Aromatherapy Institute, 1990.

Valnet, J., Duraffour, Lappraz, J.C. *Phytotherapy et Aromatherapie une Medecine Nouvelle.* Paris: Preses de La Renaissance, 1979.

Valnet, Jean. *The Practice of Aromatherapy.* New York: Destiny, 1980.

Wildwood, Christine. *Aromatherapy and Massage Book,* Portland, OR: National Book, 1995.

————. *Encyclopedia of Aromatherapy.* New York: Inner Traditions, 1996.

Worwood, Valerie Ann. *The Complete Book of Essential Oils and Aromatherapy, Aromantics.* London: Pan Books, 1987.

Herbs, Beauty and Perfume

Busch, Julia. *Home Guide to Natural Beauty Care*. Berkeley, CA: Berkeley Publishing Group, 1995.

Gladstar, Rosemary. *Herbal Healing for Women*. New York: Simon and Schuster, 1993.

Gumbel, Dietrich. *Principles of Holistic Skin Therapy with Herbal Essences*. Portland, OR: Karl F. Haug Publishers, 1986.

Hoffman, David. *The Holistic Herbal*. Forris, Scotland: The Findham Press, 1983.

Leigh, Michelle Domonique. *Inner Peace, Outer Beauty*. New York: Carol Publishing Group, 1995.

Maple, Eric. *The Magic of Perfume: Aromatics and Their Esoteric Significance*. York Beach, ME: Samuel Weiser, 1973.

Miller, Richard and Iona. *The Magical and Ritual Use of Perfumes*. New York: Destiny, 1990.

Rechelbacher, Horst. *Rejuvenation: A Wellness Guide for Women and Men*. Wellingborough, England: Thorsons, 1987.

Rose, Jeanne. *Kitchen Cosmetics*. Berkeley, CA: North Atlantic Books, 1988.

———. *Jeanne Rose's Modern Herbal*. New York: Grosset and Dunlap, 1987.

Tenny, Louise. *Today's Herbal Health*. Woodland, 1997.

Van Toller, S. and G.H. Dodd, eds. *Perfumery. The Psychology and Biology of Frangrance.* New York: Chapman and Hall, 1988.

————. *Fragrance: The Psychology and Biology of Perfume.* New York: Elsevier Applied Science, 1992.

Minerals, Gems and Crystals

Baer, R. and V. Baer. *The Crystal Connection.* New York: Harper and Row, 1987.

Bhattacharya, A. *Gemtherapy.* Calcutta, India: Firma KLM Private LTD, 1976.

Calverly, R. *The Language of Crystals.* Toronto, Ontario: Radionics Research Association, 1986.

Johari, Harish. *The Healing Power of Gemstones.* New York: Destiny, 1988.

Klein, Hurlbut. *Manual of Mineralogy.* New York: John Wiley and Sons, 1977.

Kunz, George Frederick. *The Curious Lore of Precious Stones.* New York: Dover Publications, 1913, 1971.

Gurudas. *Gem Elixirs and Vibrational Healing.* San Rafael, CA. Cassandra Press, 1985.

Melody. *Love is in the Earth.* Earth Love Publishing House, 1991.

Raphaell, Katrina. *Crystal Healing: The Therapeutic Application of Crystals and Stones.* Santa Fe, NM: Aurora Press, 1987.

Simon and Schuster's. Rocks and Minerals. New York: Simon and Schuster, 1977.

Sofianides, Anna S. and George E. Harlow. *Gems and Crystals*. New York: Simon and Schuster, 1990.

Webster, Robert. *Gems, Their Sources, Descriptions and Identification*. Butterworth and Co., 1975.

Vibrational Medicine, Color, Sound and other topics

Ardell, D. *High Level Wellness: An Alternative to Doctors, Drugs and Disease*. New York: Bantam Books, 1979.

Babbit, E. S. *The Principles of Light and Color*. New York: Citadel Press, 1967.

Becker, R. and G. Selden. *The Body Electric: Electromagnetism and the Foundaton of Life*. New York: William Morrow and Co., 1985.

Brennan, Barbara Ann. *Hands of Light*. New York: Bantam, 1989.

Clark, L. *The Ancient Art of Color Therapy*. New York: Pocket Books, 1975.

Chopra, Deepak, M.D. *Quantum Healing*. New York: Bantam, 1989.

David, W. *The Harmonics of Sound, Color and Vibration: A System for Self-Awareness and Soul Evolution*. DeVorss and Co., 1980.

————. *Fragrant and Radiant Healing Symphony.* Sussex, England: Academy of the Science of Man, 1949.

Garfield, Leah Maggie. *Sound Medicine.* New Orleans, LA: Celestial Arts, 1987.

Gerber, Richard. *Vibrational Medicine.* Santa Fe, NM: Bear and Company, 1988.

Gimbel, T. *Healing Through Color.* Saffron Walden, England: C. W. Daniel, 1980.

Hunt, Roland. *The Seven Keys to Color Healing.* New York: Harper and Row, 1971.

Leadbeater, C.W. *The Chakras.* Wheaton, IL: Theosophical Publishing House, 1977.

Liberman, Jacob. *Light: Medicine of the Future.* Santa Fe, NM: Bear and Comapny, 1993.

MacIvor, V., S. LaForest. *Vibrations: Healing Through Color Homeopathy and Radionics.* York Beach, ME: Samuel Weiser, 1979.

Myss, Carolyn. *Anatomy of a Spirit.* New York: Random House, 1997.

Oldfield, H., R. Coghill. *The Dark Side of the Brain.* Shaftesbury, Dorset: Element, 1988.

Ouseley, S. G. J. *The Power of the Rays.* L. N. Fowler and Co., 1986.

Powell, A. E. *The Etheric Double: The Health Aura of Man.* Wheaton, IL: Theosophical Publishing House, 1969.

Siegel, B. *Love, Medicine and Miracles.* New York: Harper and Row, 1986.

Summer Rain, Mary. *Earthway: A Native American Visionary Path to Total Mind, Body and Spirit Health.* New York: Pocket Books, 1993.

Tiller, W. "Some Energy Field Observations of Man and Nature." *The Kirlian Aura.* New York: Anchor Press, 1974.

Sources

Find below, in alphabetical order, some of the recommended labels of essential oils for aromatherapy use, found in health-food stores and other retail sources:

Aroma Care, O.S.A.	Osmosis, Canada
Aromaland	Primavera Life
Aroma Vera	Simplers
Oshadhi	Tisserand Aromatherapy

Aromatherapy Education

Academy of Aromatherapy
Lake Kotecha, Ontario, Canada
Telephone: 519-885-OILS

Aroma Botanica Institute
Christ J. Ubuchowsky, New Mexico
Telephone: 505-984-1874

Aromatherapy Institute and Research
Victoria Edwards, California
Telephone: 916-965-7546

Michael Scholes School of Aromatic Studies
Micheal Scholes and Joan Clark, California
Telephone: 800-677-2368 or 310-276-1191

National Association for Holistic Aromatherapy
Jeanne Rose, California
Telephone: 800-566-6735

Pacific Institute of Aromatherapy
Kurt Schanaubelt, California
Telephone: 415-459-3998

The Tisserand Institute
Robert Tisserand, England
Telephone: 0273-206640 / 772479

Aromatherapy Publications

Aromatherapy Quarterly
5 Ranelagh Ave
London SW13 OBY England
in USA: P.O. Box 421
Inverness, CA 94937-0421

AAOA: New Quarterly
P.O. Box 309
Depoe Bay, OR 97341
Internet: www.aaoa.org

The Aromatic Thymes
18-4 East Dundee Road, Suite 200
Barrington, IL 60010
email: aromatic@interaccess.com

NAHA: Scentsitivity
P.O. Box 17622
Boulder, CO 80308
Internet: www.weskimo.com/~hhnews/naha

The International Journal of Aromatherapy
In USA:
P.O. Box 309
Depoe Bay, OR 97341
Internet: www.aaoa.org
in the U.K.: P.O. Box 746
Hove, East Sussex, BN3 3XA, England

Organizations

Canadian Federation of Aromatherapists
P.O. Box 68571-1235
Williams Parkway East
Bramalea, Ontario L6S 6A1 Canada

International Federation of Aromatherapists
46 Dalkeith Rd., Dulwich
London SE21 8LS
England

National Association for Holistic Aromatherapy (NAHA)
P.O. Box 17622
Boulder, CO 80308-7622 U.S.A.

The Association of Tisserand Aromatherapists
44 Ditchling Rise
Brighton, E. Sussex BNI 3PY
England

Index

Abdominal gas, 149

Aching muscles, 149

Acne, 23–24, 42, 113,
117–119, 121,
125–128, 132,
135–138

Almond, 99, 118, 124,
132, 135, 137–140,
153

Aloe vera, 99, 119,
133–134, 141–142,
153

Amethyst, 228

Analgesic, 38, 41, 45, 51,
58, 64, 89

Anti-allergic, 42

Anti-bactericide, 85

Anti-fungal, 85

Anti-inflammatory, 42, 137

Anti-oxidant, 122,
125–126

Anti-phlogistic, 82

Anti-stress, 58

Anti-viral, 45, 85

Antibiotic, 26

Antiseptic, 23, 26, 38, 48,
51, 55, 58, 61, 67, 82,
85, 89, 124, 128, 146

Antispasmodic, 35, 41–42,
54, 64, 76, 79, 89

Anxiety, 67, 158

Aphrodisiac, 53–54, 68,
71–72, 82, 89

Aquamarine, 204, 212, 228

Asthma, 41, 43, 64, 215

Astringent, 48, 51, 72, 89,
113, 124, 127, 136

Athlete's foot, 149

Avocado, 99, 134, 141

Bactericide, 59, 123

Base notes, 102–103

Basil, 32–35, 49, 75, 103,
127, 148, 153–155,
157, 227

Bergamot, 23, 32, 36–38,
103, 147–148,
154–156, 227

Beryl, 227
Black currant seed, 119–120
Bladder infections, 149–150
Blemished skin, 117, 128
Body odor, 177–179
Boils, 150
Borage Oil, 120
Brewers yeast, 120, 130–131
Bronchitis, 33, 45, 64, 76
Bruises, 42
Burns, 43, 58, 119, 149

Cancer, 194
Chakras, 208, 222
Chamomile, 32, 39–42, 103, 124,
    126–127, 129–132, 134–135,
    137, 139, 142, 148–150,
    153–155, 157, 204–205
Cinnamon, 23
Citrine, 227
Clary sage, 33, 39, 77–79, 103,
    126–127, 130, 135, 148, 153,
    227
Clove, 23
Colds, 64, 76, 157
Comfrey, 121, 127, 132, 137–138
Congested sinuses, 150
Cosmetics, 3–4, 6, 23, 65, 82, 93,
    110, 117, 126, 142

Coughs, 33, 64
Crystals, 42, 194–198, 202,
    210–217, 219, 221–222,
    224–225
Cumin, 23

Decongestant, 76, 124, 147
Deodorant, 38, 55
Dermatosis, 42
Diamond, 198, 200, 209,
    224–226, 228
Diarrhea, 68, 82, 151, 157
Digestive, 42, 67–68, 76, 89, 122,
    127, 145, 155, 162, 227
Digestive system, 42, 76, 145,
    155, 162, 227
Dyspepsia, 42

Eczema, 51, 71
Emerald, 137, 213, 227
Emotion, 18, 20, 24–25, 58, 98,
    162, 184, 187
Enzymes, 122, 124, 127
Esters, 7
Eucalyptus, 10, 32, 43–45, 59, 63,
    126, 148, 150–151
Evening primrose oil, 122, 124,
    134
Expectorant, 45, 64, 82, 85, 90

Facials, 113, 117
Female organs, 38, 51
Fennel, 22
Flatulence, 64, 76, 157
Flu, 33, 61, 151, 157
Food poisoning, 151
Fragrance, 10, 15, 38, 49, 59, 63,
    79, 82, 93, 101, 167
Frankincense, 32, 46–48, 103,
    126, 134, 148, 227–228

Garnet, 220, 227
Gastro-intestinal, 42
Geranium, 11, 32–33, 37, 39,
    49–51, 59, 83, 103, 126, 141,
    148, 151, 153, 227
Grapeseed, 99, 134

Hair treatment, 101, 141
Hazelnut, 99, 134, 142
Heart, 67–68, 71, 81, 94, 161,
    165, 169, 214–215, 219, 221,
    227
Hemostatic, 51, 61, 72, 90
Herpes simplex, 45, 151
Honey, 112–113, 121, 123–124,
    130–133, 139–140, 151, 156
Hormones, 7, 23, 51
Hypotensive, 61, 148
Hyssop, 22

Immune System, 7, 21, 214, 217
Indole, 53, 65
Infant massage oil, 142
Inflammation, 21, 89, 125, 212
Insect, 33, 35, 51, 149
Insomnia, 58, 68, 152, 157, 210
Irritation, 21, 156

Jade, black, 149, 223, 227
Jasmine, 32, 39, 52–54, 65, 103,
    126, 227–228
Jojoba, 99, 141, 153
Juniper, 23, 37

Lavender, 10, 25–27, 32–33, 37,
    39, 43, 49, 55–59, 63, 75, 83,
    103, 124, 126–127, 130–132,
    134–135, 140–142, 147–150,
    152–155, 157–158, 166,
    188–189, 210, 228
Lemon, 24, 32, 43, 59–61, 63, 67,
    75, 103, 126, 131, 133, 135,
    137, 146–148, 150–151,
    154–155, 157, 227
Lime, 33
Love, 71, 95, 136, 187, 190,
    193–194, 204, 210, 218
Lungs, 48, 64, 90, 145, 171, 228

Masks, 48, 112, 115, 122, 125, 136
Massage, 15, 18–20, 45, 53, 58, 64, 76, 99, 101, 111, 142, 145, 148–149, 153, 170, 175
Meditation, 81, 175, 178
Memory, 9, 20, 24–25, 76, 89, 96, 102, 161–163, 173, 177, 184–185, 188–189, 210
Menstruation, 49
Mental fatigue, 64, 152
Menthol, 63
Mint, peppermint, 32, 62–64, 75, 126–127, 131, 137, 141, 148–149, 152–153, 155, 157–158
Moisturize, 111–113, 117, 121
Motion sickness, 153, 157
Mugwort, 22
Mustard, 22

Nasal, 24, 76, 178
Nausea, 35, 153, 157
Neroli, 14, 32, 39, 59, 65, 67–68, 103, 124, 126, 130, 134, 139–140, 148, 153–155, 158, 166, 175, 228
Nervous system, 19, 41, 51, 54–55, 79, 90, 146, 208–209, 217, 228

Nervous tension, 158
Nut butters, 112, 124

Odor, 33, 42–43, 47, 49, 57, 63, 71, 95, 101–102, 162–163, 165, 177–179
Orange blossom, 14, 32, 65–68, 174, 176, 227–228
Oregano, 23, 150

Parasites, 41
Pennyroyal, 22
Peppermint, 32, 62–64, 75, 126–127, 131, 137, 141, 148–149, 152–153, 155, 157–158
Perfume, 3, 47, 57, 71–72, 81, 93–94, 99, 101, 104–105, 173, 190
Perfumery, 25, 33, 41, 43, 54, 65, 72, 82, 87, 102
Photo-sensitive, 147
Piezoeletricity, 196
Pine, 23, 83
PMS, 153, 158
Preparation, teas, 154

Rancidity, 13, 99, 120
Rashes, 42, 118–119, 135

Respiratory infections, 76, 82, 150, 157

Respiratory system, 64, 146

Rheumatism, 76, 211

Rose, 11, 14, 32, 49, 59, 69–73, 81, 103, 124, 126–127, 130–131, 134–136, 140, 148, 151, 154–155, 158, 166, 170, 218, 227

Rose hip oil, 134

Rose quartz, 218, 227

Rosemary, 32, 43, 63, 74–76, 103, 111, 113, 126–127, 129, 133, 137, 141, 147–148, 150, 152, 228

Rue, 22

Rutilated quartz, 216–217, 227

Sage, clary, 33, 39, 77–79, 103, 126–127, 130, 135, 148, 153, 227

Sandalwood, 7, 32, 49, 59, 72, 77, 80–82, 103, 126, 134, 139, 148, 153, 227–228

Sapphire, 211, 228

Sassafras, 23

Savory, 23, 150

Scarring, 26

Scrub, 113, 129–133

Seaweed, 112, 125

Sedative, 38, 41, 48, 54, 58, 67, 72, 79, 82, 88, 90, 146, 166

Sensation, sensitivity, 18, 21, 23, 148, 177, 198

Sesame, 99, 124, 131

Sexual, 25, 71, 88, 177–178, 220–221, 227

Shock, 25, 41, 67

Skin, 12, 19–21, 23–24, 33, 37, 42–43, 48, 58, 71, 82, 90, 94–95, 100, 109–113, 115, 117–140, 145, 147–148, 150, 153

Slippery elm, 125, 137–139

Soil, 8, 65, 98, 201

Sound, 187, 193, 206–207, 227–228

Spasm, 35, 67, 88

Spirulina, 125, 137–138

Stimulant, 35, 45, 51, 76, 88, 90, 124, 212

Stress, 6, 19, 23, 67, 177

Suppository, 145, 149, 151

Swelling, 42, 120

Tea, 32, 53, 67, 76–77, 83–85, 103, 112, 117, 126, 130–133, 137, 147–158

Tea tree, 32, 83–85, 103, 126, 133, 137, 147–151, 154–157

Teething, 42
Thyme, 22, 150
Tonic, 42, 54, 61, 79, 88, 90, 124
Topaz, 227
Tourmaline, 172, 199, 213–214, 220, 222, 227–228
Toxic, Toxicity, 19–23, 146

Ulcers, 42
Urinary system, 227
Uterine, 72, 90, 153
Uterine cramps, 153

Vegetable oils, 12–13, 16, 98–99, 141
Viruses, 8, 27
Vitamin E, 98–99, 113, 120, 126, 134, 139, 151–152

Wintergreen, 22
Wormwood, 22
Wounds, 43, 48, 90

Yeast, 112, 120, 130–131
Ylang ylang, 14, 32, 86–88, 103, 148

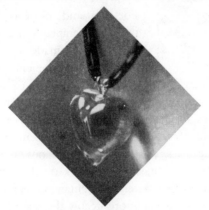

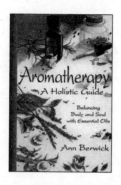